SAQs for the Final FRCA

SAQs for the Final FRCA

James Shorthouse MBBS BSc(Hons) FRCA
Specialty Registrar in Anaesthesia
Oxford Deanery

Graham Barker MBBS BSc(Hons) FRCA
Specialty Registrar in Anaesthesia
Oxford Deanery

Carl Waldmann MA MB,BChir FRCA EDIC
Consultant in Anaesthesia and Intensive Care
Royal Berkshire Hospital
Reading

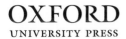

OXFORD
UNIVERSITY PRESS

OXFORD
UNIVERSITY PRESS

Great Clarendon Street, Oxford OX2 6DP
United Kingdom

Oxford University Press is a department of the University of Oxford.
It furthers the University's objective of excellence in research, scholarship,
and education by publishing worldwide. Oxford is a registered trade mark of
Oxford University Press in the UK and in certain other countries

British Library Cataloguing in Publication Data
Data available

Library of Congress Cataloging in Publication Data
Data available

ISBN 978-0-19-958328-7

Printed and bound by CPI Group (UK) Ltd, Croydon, CR0 4YY

James Shorthouse

To Abby, Charlie, and my family for all their love, help, and support.

Graham Barker

To Gemma, Joseph, and my parents and family for their
help, advice, love, and support over the years.

Carl Waldmann

To Tanya, Anna, Mia, and Felicity for their patience.

Foreword

The Short Answer Question section of the Final FRCA written paper is likely to be quite dissimilar to any examination the candidate has attempted previously. It is extremely time-pressured and mentally exhausting and it requires concise, relevant answers provided in a structured, legible manner. It is often the making or breaking of a candidate!

This book provides model answers to a wide range of topics within the Final FRCA examination syllabus. The model answers contain abundant line diagrams, and these are suitable for use in the examination. Similarly, the style of the answers is in bullet-points and concise statements of fact; such presentation is not only ideal for use in the examination, but provides a comfortable medium for reading and learning.

The authors place emphasis on topical issues, which have traditionally been difficult to study. Lists of resources provide further detail about these, allowing the reader to make sure they are aware of the myriad of issues facing the modern anaesthetist.

The authors' obvious passion for education shines through in this book as they bring their detailed knowledge of the subject and the examination to bear. Succinct, clear, and relevant, this book is clearly the result of many hours of dedicated work. Although many examination preparation texts have been produced for medicine and anaesthesia, this new text brings a unique, welcome, and refreshing approach, and I wholeheartedly recommend it to candidates facing the Final FRCA examination.

I commend the authors on an excellent text and wish all the readers the best as they prepare for this crucial exam.

Jonathan G Hardman

Editor, British Journal of Anaesthesia

Associate Professor and Reader in Anaesthesia, University of Nottingham

Honorary Consultant Anaesthetist, University Hospitals NHS Trust, Nottingham

Acknowledgements

We would like to thank the following people for their help, advice, and input in writing this textbook:

Dr Simon Berg

Dr Manish Bhardwaj

Dr Bob Bingham

Dr Peter Cole

Dr Chris Danbury

Dr Niamh Feely

Dr Svetlana Galitzine

Dr David Garry

Dr David Goldhill

Dr John Griffiths

Dr Elaine Hill

Dr Andrew Kitching

Dr Sara McDouall

Dr Peter Merjavy

Mandy Odell

Dr Simon Raby

Dr Matthew Rowland

Dr Robin Russell

Professor Andrew Shorthouse

Dr Neil Soni

Dr Mhairi Speirs

Dr Jon Westbrook

Contents

Abbreviations

1°	primary
2°	secondary
↑	increased
↓	decreased
AAA	abdominal aortic aneurysm
A–a	alveolar–arterial
AAFB	acid- and alcohol-fast bacillus
AAGBI	Association of Anaesthetists of Great Britain & Ireland
ABC	airway, breathing, circulation
ABG	arterial blood gas
ACE	angiotensin-converting enzyme
ACh	acetylcholine
ACS	abdominal compartment syndrome
ADH	antidiuretic hormone
AFOI	awake fibreoptic intubation
AKA	above-knee amputation
ALI	acute lung injury
ALP	alkaline phosphatase
ALT	alanine aminotransferase
ANS	autonomic nervous system
AP	anteroposterior
APAGBI	Association of Paediatric Anaesthetists of Great Britain & Ireland
APTT	activated partial thromboplastin time
AR	aortic regurgitation
ARDS	adult respiratory distress syndrome
ARF	acute renal failure
AS	aortic stenosis
ASIS	anterior superior iliac spine
AST	aspartate aminotransferase
ATLS	Advanced Trauma and Life Support
ATP	anti-tachycardia pacing
AVR	aortic valve replacement
AV	atrioventricular (heart)
BBB	blood–brain barrier
BD, bid	twice daily
BKA	below-knee amputation
BMI	body mass index
BNF	British National Formulary
BP	blood pressure
C1–7	cervical vertebrae 1–7
CABG	coronary artery bypass graft
CHF	congestive heart failure
CIM	critical illness myopathy
CIN	contrast-induced nephropathy
CIP	critical illness polyneuropathy
CMAP	compound muscle action potential

CME	Continuing Medical Education
$CMRO_2$	cerebral metabolic oxygen consumption
CNS	central nervous system
CO	cardiac output
CO_2	carbon dioxide
COPD	chronic obstructive pulmonary disease
CPAP	continuous positive airway pressure
CPB	cardiopulmonary bypass
CPET	cardiopulmonary exercise testing
CPR	cardiopulmonary resuscitation
CPSP	chronic post-surgical pain
CRF	chronic renal failure
CRP	C-reactive protein
CRPS	complex regional pain syndrome
CRT	capillary refill time
CSE	combined spinal–epidural
CSF	cerebrospinal fluid
CSWS	cerebral salt-wasting syndrome
CT	computed tomography
CTG	cardiotocograph
CVA	cerebrovascular accident
CVP	central venous pressure
CVS	cardiovascular system
CVVH	continuous venovenous haemodialysis
CXR	chest X-ray
DI	diabetes insipidus
DIC	disseminated intravascular coagulation
DM	diabetes mellitus
DPG	diphosphoglycerate
DVT	deep vein thrombosis
ECG	electrocardiogram
ECMO	extracorporeal membrane oxygenation
EEG	electroencephalogram
ENT	ear, nose, and throat
ERCP	endoscopic retrograde cholangiopancreatography
Et	end-tidal gas
ETT	endotracheal tube
EVAR	endovascular aneurysm repair
FBC	full blood count
FFP	fresh frozen plasma
Fi	fraction of inspired gas
FRC	functional residual capacity
GA	general anaesthesia
GBS	Guillain–Barré syndrome
GCS	Glasgow Coma Scale
G&S	group and save
GFR	glomerular filtration rate
GI	gastrointestinal
GORD	gastro-oesophageal reflux disease
GTN	glyceryl trinitrate
GU	genitourinary

Hb	haemoglobin
HDU	high dependency unit
HME	heat–moisture exchange
HPV	hypoxic pulmonary vasoconstriction
HR	heart rate
HRT	hormone replacement therapy
IABP	intra-aortic balloon pump
ICP	intracranial pressure
ICS	intra-operative cell salvage
ICU	intensive care unit (PICU, paediatric ICU)
IHD	ischaemic heart disease
IJV	internal jugular vein
ILMA	intubating laryngeal mask airway
IM	intramuscular
IOP	intraocular pressure
IPPV	intermittent positive pressure ventilation
IV	intravenous
IVC	inferior vena cava
IVRA	intravenous regional anaesthesia
JVP	jugular venous pressure
L1–5	lumbar vertebrae 1–5
LA	local anaesthetic
LDH	lactate dehydrogenase
LFT	liver function test
LMA	laryngeal mask airway
LMWH	low molecular weight heparin
LP	lumbar puncture
LRTI	lower respiratory tract infection
LSCS	lower segment Caesarean section
LV	left ventricle
LVEDP	left ventricular end-diastolic pressure
MAOI	monoamine oxidase inhibitor
MAP	mean arterial pressure
MC&S	microscopy, culture, and sensitivity
mcg	microgram
MI	myocardial infarction
MIBG	meta-iodobenzylguanidine
MR	mitral regurgitation
MRI	magnetic resonance imaging
MS	mitral stenosis
MVR	mitral valve replacement
N_2O	nitrous oxide
NG, NGT	nasogastric (tube)
NBM	nil by mouth
NDMB	non-depolarizing muscle blocker
NIBP	non-invasive blood pressure
NICE	National Institute for Health and Clinical Excellence
NIV	non-invasive ventilation
NMDA	N-methyl-D-aspartate
NPSA	National Patient Safety Agency
NSAID	non-steroidal anti-inflammatory drug

O_2	oxygen
OCD	obsessive-compulsive disorder
OCP	oral contraceptive pill
ODP	operating department practitioner
OETT	oral endotracheal tube (COETT, cuffed OETT)
OSA	obstructive sleep apnoea
PA	pulmonary artery
PAC	pulmonary artery catheter
PAP	pulmonary artery pressure
$PaCO_2$	partial pressure of arterial carbon dioxide
PaO_2	partial pressure of arterial oxygen
PCA	patient-controlled analgesia
PCR	polymerase chain reaction
PDPH	post-dural puncture headache
PE	pulmonary embolism
PEEP	positive end-expiratory pressure
PFT	pulmonary function test
PgI_2	prostacyclin
PICU	paediatric intensive care unit
PNS	peripheral nervous system
PO	by mouth
PONV	postoperative nausea and vomiting
PPE	personnel protective equipment
PR	per rectum
PRC	packed red cells
PRN	as required
PT	prothrombin time
PVC	premature ventricular contraction
$PvCO_2$	partial pressure of venous CO_2
PVD	peripheral vascular disease
PVR	pulmonary vascular resistance
qds	four times daily
RA	regional anaesthesia
RAE	Ring, Adair, and Elwyn
RCT	randomized controlled trials
RR	respiratory rate
RSI	rapid sequence induction
RV	right ventricle
SA	sinoatrial node
SAH	subarachnoid haemorrhage
SBP	systolic blood pressure
SIADH	syndrome of inappropriate antidiuretic hormone
SIRS	systemic inflammatory response syndrome
SLE	systemic lupus erythematosus
SNP	sodium nitroprusside
SOB	short of breath
SVC	superior vena cava
SVR	systemic vascular resistance
SVT	supraventricular tachycardia
T1–12	thoracic vertebrae 1–12
TB	tuberculosis

TCI	target-controlled infusion
TDS	three times daily
T_3	tri-iodothyronine
T_4	thyroxine
TAP	transversus abdominis plane
TEG	thromboelastography
TENS	transcutaneous electrical nerve stimulation
TFT	thyroid function test
TIA	transient ischaemic attack
TIVA	total intravenous anaesthesia
TKR	total knee replacement
TLC	total lung capacity
TNF	tumour necrosis factor
TOE	transoesophageal echocardiography
TPN	total parenteral nutrition
U&E	urea & electrolytes
URTI	upper respiratory tract infection
UTI	urinary tract infection
VAE	venous air embolism
VAP	ventilator-associated pneumonia
VC	vital capacity
VF	ventricular fibrillation
VSD	ventricular septal defect
VT	ventricular tachycardia
VTE	venous thromboembolism
WBC/WCC	white blood cell count
WHO	World Health Organization

Introduction

The aim of the authors is to produce a clear and concise text which will aid the Final FRCA Examination candidate in tackling the Short Answer Question (SAQ) Paper. The model answers in this textbook are relevant to a wide range of topics within the examination syllabus.

At the beginning of most questions is a short statement underlying the aim of both the question and the model answer, relevant to passing the examination and to clinical anaesthesia.

The model answers included in this text are exactly that—'model'. In some cases they contain considerably more information than is required 'just to pass' an SAQ, i.e. more than about 12 minutes of writing. Therefore candidates should not be disappointed if their practice answers are shorter than the answers in this textbook. This has been intentional as we are aiming not only to provide candidates with as detailed an answer as possible, i.e. a '2+' answer, but also to impart some factual knowledge that will aid revision for both the SAQ and SOE sections of the examination.

As well as concentrating on clinical and topical areas, we have included a detailed section on anatomy and regional techniques; we feel that anatomy is often left until last in the revision timetable as it has traditionally been the area with which candidates feel least comfortable.

Following recent correspondence with the Chair of the Final FRCA Examining Board, we have learnt that the College is placing less emphasis on the use of diagrams within SAQ answers such as anatomy and regional topics. They feel that the diagrams by past candidates have been 'poorly drawn, ambiguously labelled, and small, making them difficult to mark'. It is suggested that 'candidates use line diagrams as an *aide memoire* in their examination preparations but not include them in their answers unless explicitly asked to do so in the question'. The anatomy and regional answers in this text will contain accompanying simple line diagrams where appropriate. We feel that whilst every candidate has different styles and methods of revision, the use of visual schematics and line diagrams is still the best way to learn concepts, especially in anatomy and regional techniques. Candidates must ensure that if they do produce diagrams in the actual examination, they are legible, clear, large, and well labelled.

We have deliberately avoided including basic science SAQs in this text as we feel that they are already adequately covered in previous texts of a similar nature. This has allowed us to concentrate fully on more clinical/topical issues. It should be emphasized that basic science SAQs do appear in this section of the paper and must not be ignored by the candidate.

More recently, the Royal College of Anaesthetists has placed greater emphasis on testing the candidate's knowledge of topical issues, recent guidelines, and public interest subjects relevant to anaesthesia, critical care, and pain medicine within the written paper. These are often not subjects which may have been thought about by the candidate; for example, a recent question asked about the relevance of child abuse to anaesthesia. We have incorporated both topical issues and questions on recent guidelines from the Association of Anaesthetists, NICE, WHO, and NPSA, to name but a few, into our text in order to give the candidate the most accurate and up-to-date revision aid that we can. A list of online resources to locate these topical issues and guidelines is included at the end of this introduction.

We want to expose Final FRCA Examination candidates to the range of topics used within the written paper, the style and layout required, and the use of diagrams/pictures, such that they will feel more confident when sitting the paper. The text may be used by tutors or consultants when providing structured informal or formal teaching for the examination.

We also envisage our textbook providing an additional resource for the Structured Oral Examination (SOE) as there is a significant amount of crossover between the two sections of the examination.

About the Final FRCA Examination

The written part of the Final FRCA Examination is currently a stand-alone section which the candidate is required to pass successfully before attempting the SOE. At the time of writing, it is divided into two papers with marks from both sections combined to produce a single result for the written section:

- A 3 hour paper consisting of 60 multiple true/false questions (MCQs) and 30 single best-answer questions (SBAs). The MCQ–SBA section is beyond the scope of this book and is not discussed any further.
- A 3 hour paper consisting of twelve SAQs. All questions carry equal marking, but pass marks may vary from question to question and are decided by the Examiners' Committee, using modified Angoff referencing, during paper-setting sessions.

Each section carries equal weighting.

Currently, the candidate is provided with a question sheet containing all 12 questions (including mark allocation percentages), scrap paper for notes/planning, and six different coloured booklets in which to answer the questions:

- Questions 1 and 2 in the Blue Book A
- Questions 3 and 4 in the Pink Book B
- Questions 5 and 6 in the Green Book C
- Questions 7 and 8 in the Yellow Book D
- Questions 9 and 10 in the Orange Book E
- Questions 11 and 12 in the Grey Book F.

In these booklets, one question will be printed on the first page, and the second question will be printed half-way through the book.

It is imperative that candidates understand that they *must answer all 12 questions*. The written section will be failed if questions are omitted accidentally or on purpose, or are answered in the wrong booklet. Do not undo months of hard work and financial expense by committing clerical or organizational errors.

Techniques

Candidates often fail this section of the written paper not through lack of knowledge, but because of lack of organization in both pre-examination revision and structure whilst attempting the SAQ paper. We cannot emphasize strongly enough the importance of *time management* when writing this paper.

This written paper is unlike any other that the candidate has attempted previously; it is extremely time-pressured, mentally exhausting, and requires concise and relevant answers in a structured and legible manner. Thus it is vital that the candidate develops a technique to suit his/her writing style so that the whole SAQ paper can be completed successfully within the allotted time limit. The only way to achieve this is by practising past SAQ examinations repeatedly. Not only will this allow the candidate to build up the stamina required to concentrate for 3 hours and answer all the questions, but it will also allow him/her to practice planning for the questions, drawing simple line diagrams rapidly, and structuring the question clearly and legibly

The technique of answering questions will vary between candidates. No more than *15 minutes* should be spent on each question, despite the temptation to overrun on strong topics and leave weaker topics to the end with less answering time. This is usually divided into 2–3 minutes planning and 12–13 minutes writing.

Suggested methods of time-allocation are as follows.

a) Spend approximately 35 minutes at the beginning reading the question carefully and producing a short plan or spider-diagram/mind-map for each question. Once all plans are completed, this leaves 2 hours and 25 minutes to produce answers for the 12 questions, or 12 minutes per question.

b) Spend a minute reading through the paper and deciding what order to answer the questions (take great care with answering the right question in the right booklet if altering the natural order of the paper!), then making a plan, and then answering the question for that plan.

c) Although planning the question is recommended, some (lucky) candidates have the ability to do this in their head, and therefore will be able to allocate 15 minutes per question solely for writing.

General hints

- From March 2011, all SAQs will be marked out of 20; the awarding of 10% of the marks for clarity, judgement and prioritizing *has been scrapped.*
- Make it easy for the examiner who has to mark hundreds of versions of the same question over a few nights; ensure that you practise legible handwriting and appropriate spelling.
- Use bullet points rather than large chunks of prose text; remember to leave a blank line between paragraphs or sections to demonstrate clearly a new part of the answer. Again, this is for the marker's sake.
- When instructed to do so, produce a large well-labelled simple line diagram. Use a sharpened pencil with a rubber for corrections rather than pen, as diagrams often become indecipherable following pen corrections and this only serves to irritate the marker.
- Make sure that answers are relevant. Do not waste valuable time producing facts which do not answer the question. For instance, when answering a question on the intravenous fluid management of a dehydrated child, listing the methods of assessing dehydration in a child is not relevant unless specifically asked for in a question stem, and will not gain any marks.

Resources

Website links for useful sources of revision for the SAQ section of the examination are listed below.

- Royal College of Anaesthetists publications: http://www.rcoa.ac.uk/index.asp?PageID=57
- *Continuing Education in Anaesthesia, Critical Care, and Pain* articles: http://ceaccp.oxfordjournals.org/archive/
- *British Journal of Anaesthesia* review articles: http://bja.oxfordjournals.org/archive/
- Association of Anaesthetists guidelines: http://www.aagbi.org/publications/guidelines.htm
- *Anaesthesia* review articles: http://www3.interscience.wiley.com/journal/119877700/issue
- NICE guidelines: http://www.nice.org.uk/Guidance/Date
- NPSA guidelines: http://www.npsa.nhs.uk/nrls/alerts-and-directives/
- NCEPOD Reports: http://www.ncepod.org.uk/reports.htm
- British Pain Society guidelines: http://www.britishpainsociety.org/pub_professional.htm
- Association of Paediatric Anaesthetists guidelines: http://www.apagbi.org.uk/index.asp?PageID=6
- Update in Anaesthesia: http://www.nda.ox.ac.uk/wfsa/html/pages/up_issu.htm
- Instant Anatomy: http://www.instantanatomy.net/
- New York School of Regional Anesthesia: http://www.nysora.com/

Finally

- Eat and sleep well the night before!
- Try not to panic. Part of this examination is about keeping a cool head.
- Bring nice pens, plus spares and a pencil for diagrams.
- Plan your journey to the venue and leave time to spare.
- Arrive early and bring photo ID as told.
- Read the questions (properly).
- Write legibly and space answers out. Make it easy for the examiner!
- Don't overrun on questions.
- Good luck from us!

Part 1 **Clinical Anaesthesia**

Chapter 1: **General Anaesthesia**

Q1 Airway Anaesthesia

You wish to perform an awake fibreoptic intubation on a 24-year-old man who is listed for open reduction and internal fixation of his fractured left mandible.

a) Describe the different topical methods of anaesthetising his airway (8 marks)

b) What regional adjunct techniques may be employed? (12 marks)

Aims

Thorough topicalization of the airway will be critical to improving patient comfort and compliance during the procedure, increasing success rates with this core airway skill.

a) Pharmacological Anaesthesia

- For all topical methods, it is important to ensure that the toxic dose of LA is not exceeded
- 2% lidocaine gel or 4% or 10% lidocaine spray are applied directly to the nose and mouth (specifically the back of the tongue and the oropharynx)
- Ribbon gauze, soaked in 5% cocaine or lidocaine–phenylephrine mixture, is packed into the nasal cavity
- A mucosal atomizer device or adapted cannula attached to an oxygen supply can be used to spray LA into the nasal or oral cavity
- 'Spray-as-you-go' technique during the fibreoptic procedure via a side port on the fibreoptic scope:
  - a 16G epidural catheter, with a 2ml syringe attached to a Luer Lock connection, is threaded down the port and used for direct airway mucosal LA application
- Use of nebulized lidocaine (may require additional 'spray-as-you-go' LA)

b) Regional Anaesthesia

i) Anterior Glossopharyngeal Nerve Block
   - Patient in sitting position facing anaesthetist
   - Mouth opened widely and tongue retracted to the opposite side of the injection
   - Identify U- or J-shape made by palatoglossal arch from base of the palate to lateral margin of the tongue; injection point is 0.5cm from the lateral margin of the tongue at the floor of the mouth
   - Using a 25G spinal needle, first aspirate (if air, then withdraw superficially; if blood, redirect medially) and then inject 2ml 2% lidocaine and repeat on the opposite side

ii) External Superior Laryngeal Nerve Block
   - Patient in sitting position facing anaesthetist
   - Identify the superior cornu of the hyoid bone (beneath the angle of the mandible and medial to the carotid artery)
   - Identify the superior cornu of the thyroid cartilage by palpating along the superior border of the cartilage until just inferior to the superior cornu of the hyoid bone
   - Walk a 25G needle anteriorly and superiorly along the superior cornu of the thyroid cartilage, aiming to the lower third of the thyrohyoid membrane
   - A 'give' will indicate introduction through the membrane
   - Aspirate (if air, then withdraw superficially; if blood, redirect), and inject 2ml 2% lidocaine with 1:200,000 adrenaline; repeat on the other side

iii) Translaryngeal Anaesthesia
  - Patient in supine position with neck extended
  - Once the skin is clean and prepared, identify the cricothyroid membrane and apply a bleb of LA to the skin
  - Stabilize the trachea and insert a 20G cannula caudally, whilst aspirating for air
  - Once in the trachea, advance the cannula and remove the needle; inject 3–4ml 4% lidocaine
  - Patient will cough and disperse LA up to the vocal cords and down to the carina

Notes

Reference

Popat M, Rai M. Awake fibreoptic intubation. In: Popat M, ed. *Difficult Airway Management*. Oxford University Press, 2009; 70–4

Q2 Anaphylaxis

You are asked to anaesthetise a 24-year-old woman for a laparoscopic ovarian cystectomy. After induction with fentanyl, propofol, and atracurium, her BP measures 52/33mmHg and HR is 125bpm.

a) What other signs and symptoms may be present if anaphylaxis has occurred? (6 marks)

b) Outline i) the immediate (6 marks) and ii) the late (8 marks) management of anaphylaxis in this patient

Aims

This is core knowledge for all anaesthetists and is classic examination fodder in both the written and the clinical section. There should be no room for error in your management

a) Signs and Symptoms

- CVS compromise or collapse may be the only sign: hypotension, tachycardia, bradycardia, arrhythmia, and ultimately cardiac arrest
- Difficult to ventilate, high peak airway pressures, bronchospasm, desaturation
- Flushing, rash, urticaria
- Facial swelling, angio-oedema

b) Management

i) Immediate Management
   - Every anaesthetic department should have an 'anaphylaxis drill'
   - Stop administration of any potentially causative agents and call for help
   - Secure the airway with a tracheal tube and ventilate the lungs with 100% O_2
   - Lie the patient supine with legs elevated and secure wide-bore IV access
   - If cardiac arrest, commence CPR according to the Advanced Life Support protocol
   - Administer 50mcg (0.5ml of 1:10000 solution) IV adrenaline over 1 minute; in CVS collapse, consider an adrenaline infusion
   - For additional CVS support, consider other IV vasopressors (e.g. metaraminol or vasopressin)
   - Commence a rapid infusion of IV crystalloid (e.g. Hartmann's solution)
   - Once clinically stable, arrange transfer to ICU

ii) Late Management
   - Corticosteroids: 200mg IV hydrocortisone slowly
   - Antihistamine: 10mg IV chlorphenamine slowly
   - Bronchodilator therapy (e.g. salbutamol) if evidence of bronchospasm. Consider IV infusion if resistant bronchospasm. IV magnesium or aminophylline may also be used
   - Take mast cell tryptase samples:
     - immediately after treatment (although resuscitation must not be delayed)
     - 1–2 hours after reaction (at peak of anaphylactic reaction)
     - 24 hours post-reaction or at a later date to assess baseline tryptase levels
   - Accurate record-keeping, critical incident reporting, and clear documentation for future anaesthetics
   - The patient will require debriefing and counselling once conscious
   - Write a letter to the GP; the patient may require a MedicAlert bracelet

- Report the reaction to Committee on Safety of Medicines and fill out a BNF 'Yellow Card'
- Notify the AAGBI National Anaesthetic Anaphylaxis Database (http://www.aagbi.org)
- Refer the patient to a defined regional allergy centre:
  - skin-prick testing: shows presence of IgE antibodies
  - intradermal skin testing, if negative skin-prick test
  - serum IgE antibody assays (e.g. suxamethonium)
  - radio-allergosorbent test (RAST)
  - basophil stimulation tests: flow cytometry detects CD63 and CD203c proteins expressed on basophils during anaphylaxis (experimental)

Notes

Reference

AAGBI. *Suspected Anaphylactic Reactions Associated with Anaesthesia*, AAGBI Safety Guideline. London: AAGBI, 2009

Q3 Ankylosing Spondylitis

A 69-year-old man is listed for an elective right total hip replacement. Relevant past medical history includes long-standing ankylosing spondylitis.

a) **List the drugs available to treat ankylosing spondylitis, highlighting their adverse effects with relevance to the conduct of anaesthesia (9 marks)**

b) **What important anaesthetic considerations should be made for this case regarding the clinical features of ankylosing spondylitis? (11 marks)**

Aims

This question explores your understanding not only of the anaesthetic implications of ankylosing spondylitis, but also of the extended pharmacology and possible consequences of both common and less regularly used medications which are proving increasingly popular.

a) Pharmacological Treatments

i) NSAIDs
- Used for anti-inflammatory properties and symptomatic relief
- GI symptoms (e.g. ulceration, bleeding, vomiting): may require resuscitation and RSI
- Impaired platelet function: may ↑ perioperative bleeding and influence the decision to perform regional techniques
- Renal impairment: can affect the choice of anaesthetic drugs and inhibit platelet function
- CVS disease (due to PgI_2 inhibition): ↑ risk of perioperative CVS adverse event (e.g. MI)

ii) Disease-Modifying Anti-Rheumatic Drugs
- Used for symptomatic relief of peripheral joints
- Methotrexate: pulmonary toxicity, liver cirrhosis, blood dyscrasias
- Sulfasalazine: GI symptoms as above, haematological toxicity
- Leflunomide: GI symptoms, ↑ BP, arrhythmias, immunosuppression, deranged LFTs
- Steroids: ↑ BP, osteoporosis, GI symptoms, pancreatitis, obesity, psychiatric symptoms

iii) Immunomodulation: Anti-TNF-α Drugs
- Cytokine-based drugs: either monoclocal antibodies or fusion proteins involved in alteration of inflammation/infection responses (e.g. infliximab, adalimumab, etanercept)
- General side effects: immunosuppression, especially TB (require pre-treatment screening), reactivation of chronic hepatitis B, injection site and infusion reactions, autoimmune neurological diseases (e.g. Guillain–Barré syndrome, vasculitides)

b) Clinical Features

i) Airway
- Potential for difficult intubation because of cervical spine and temporo-mandibular joint involvement
- Risk of significant atlanto-axial subluxation, neurological damage, vertebro-basilar insufficiency during airway instrumentation and turning or moving the patient: important to maintain manual in-line stabilization during airway manoeuvres
- Vocal cords at risk of damage due to fixation and crico-arytenoid involvement
- Consider awake fibreoptic intubation or use of alternative airway adjuncts (e.g. ILMA)

ii) Skeletal Deformities
- 'Chin-on-chest' flexion deformity may complicate airway management (e.g. intubation)

- Increased risk of spinal fractures from minimal trauma: care with transfer of patient
- Other flexion deformities or scoliosis: positioning on the operating table is difficult with increased potential for pressure sores and peripheral nerve injuries

iii) Regional Anaesthesia
- May be difficult or impossible due to bony fusion and spinal involvement
- Increased risk of epidural haematoma due to a narrowed epidural canal and NSAID use
- Intrathecal injection via the paramedian approach may be the only successful route

iv) Extra-articular

Cardiovascular System
- Increased risk of aortic regurgitation, MI, and conduction defects leading to an increased susceptibility to arrhythmias
- Preoperative ECG is mandatory; consider echocardiogram if sufficient history
- Pre-induction invasive monitoring if sufficient cardiac dysfunction

Respiratory
- Restrictive pattern due to pulmonary fibrosis and costovertebral joint involvement
- Consider preoperative ABG ± lung function tests; may need postoperative HDU/ICU

Other
- Increased risk of anterior uveitis requires attention to eye care perioperatively
- Presence of amyloidosis may increase risk of renal impairment (also exacerbated by NSAIDs); preoperative U&E levels required
- Increased risk of cauda equina syndrome, cord compression, epilepsy

Notes

Reference

Woodward LJ, Kam, PC. Ankylosing spondylitis: recent developments and anaesthetic implications. *Anaesthesia*, **64**: 540–8, 2009

Q4 Anorexia

A 27-year-old woman is listed for an open reduction and internal fixation of her right ankle. She has a BMI of 16 kg/m^2 and a past medical history of anorexia nervosa.

a) Define anorexia nervosa (4 marks)

b) Outline the physiological abnormalities that may be present in this patient and how they would affect her anaesthetic management (16 marks)

Aims

This is often an under-diagnosed problem with potentially serious adverse consequences. Putting the clues together in the preoperative assessment can reap clinical benefits.

a) Definition

- BMI ≤17.5kg/m^2 (or body weight >15% below expected)
- Characteristic behaviour: avoiding food, self-induced vomiting, purging, over-exercising, use of appetite suppressants, laxatives, and diuretics
- Additional psychological disturbances (e.g. body dysmorphia, depression, OCD)
- Endocrine dysfunction: disturbance of hypothalamic–pituitary axis, resulting in amenorrhoea and loss of libido

b) Abnormalities

i) Preoperative Investigations
- Full blood count: ↑ risk of thrombocytopenia and anaemia (2° to bone marrow suppression). Low platelet count may preclude regional anaesthesia and exacerbate surgical blood loss
- Urea and electrolytes:
  - hyponatraemia, hypokalaemia, hypochloraemia, hypomagnesaemia, metabolic alkalosis (all due to vomiting and abuse of laxatives/diuretics)
  - ↑ risk of arrhythmias necessitates preoperative electrolyte correction if abnormal
- Renal profile: function may be impaired due to ↓ GFR and proteinuria
- Blood glucose test: ↑ risk of perioperative hypoglycaemia due to starvation and impaired cortisol release
- LFTs and clotting: ↑ risk of fatty liver and cirrhosis due to starvation and substance abuse. Impaired synthetic function may preclude regional anaesthesia and worsen surgical bleeding
- All patients should have an ECG due to potential abnormalities:
  - bradycardia (2° to ↓ BMR) and ST or T-wave changes
  - arrhythmias e.g. AV block, SVT, VT
  - QT prolongation (due to drugs, electrolyte abnormalities, or starvation)
- Echocardiogram if evidence of cardiac dysfunction on history, examination, or ECG:
  - impaired LV function and contractility (due to drugs or electrolyte imbalance)
  - mitral valve prolapse is more common
- ↑ risk of aspiration pneumonitis: CXR if symptomatic or if history is suggestive

ii) Intraoperative Management
- ↑ risk of gastric dilatation and delayed gastric emptying: consider NG tube and antacid and prokinetic prophylaxis prior to induction
- Rapid sequence induction is advised in these patients

- Owing to ↑ risk of pneumothorax and pneumomediastinum, avoid high airway pressures by using pressure-control ventilation
- Invasive CVS monitoring if evidence of myocardial dysfunction
- Cautious IV fluid administration because of the risk of inducing cardiac failure if myocardial dysfunction; cardiac output monitoring may guide fluid therapy
- Aims:
  - to minimize myocardial depression (if severe, central neuraxial blockade may be unwise)
  - potential for prolonged non-depolarizing muscle relaxant action in electrolyte abnormalities necessitates neuromuscular monitoring
  - altered liver function and low albumin state can alter drug binding and metabolism
  - impaired renal function alters drug metabolism and excretion and hinders the ability to cope with large fluid shifts
- ↓ body fat and poor skin quality increases the risk of intraoperative pressure sores, nerve injuries, and damage by an arterial tourniquet. Detailed care with moving and positioning is required
- ↑ risk of perioperative hypothermia due to ↓ body fat and impaired thermoregulation requires perioperative temperature monitoring and the use of active warming devices

Notes

Reference

Denner AM, Townley SA. Anorexia nervosa: perioperative implications. *Continuing Education in Anaesthesia, Critical Care & Pain,* **9**: 61–4, 2009

Q5 Antibiotics

a) **Classify the different groups of antibiotics used in clinical practice (9 marks)**

b) **Discuss the principle of antibiotic prophylaxis including a list of pros and cons (11 marks)**

Aims

This topic is dreaded by Primary and Final FRCA candidates, despite being a daily occurrence in clinical practice. We recommend categorizing antibiotics by their mode of action.

a) Antibiotic Groups

i) Inhibition of Nucleic Acid Synthesis
   - Sulphonamides: inhibit formation of dihydropteroic acid
   - Trimethoprim: inhibits dihydrofolate reductase; high affinity with bacterial subset allows selective toxicity
   - Quinolones (e.g. ciprofloxacin): inhibit DNA-gyrase, thus preventing formation of coiled DNA
   - Nitroimidazoles (e.g. metronidazole): nitrogroup interferes with DNA production and coiling intracellularly, especially in anaerobic and protozoal organisms
   - Rifampicin: prevents conversion of DNA into RNA by inhibiting RNA polymerase enzymes

ii) Modification of Cell Wall Integrity and Synthesis
   - Contain the β-lactam ring structure that mimics the D-alanyl-D-alanine peptide chains found in bacterial walls
   - Act as a group of bactericidal antibiotics by triggering cell lysis
   - Penicillin (e.g. benzylpenicillin) was the first of this group isolated, followed by penicillin V which is orally active
   - Resistance to β-lactamases improves penetration against some organisms (e.g. flucloxacillin vs *Staphylococcus aureus*)
   - Cephalosporins have a similar mechanism of action and are grouped according to generation of production, with improved spectra of activity in more recently produced compounds
   - Carbapenems (e.g. meropenem) are highly resistant to penicillinases
   - Vancomycin inhibits peptidoglycan formation in the cell wall

iii) Inhibition of Protein Synthesis
   - Act on bacterial ribosomes to prevent reproduction and growth
   - Bacterial ribosomes are composed of a 50/30s subunit whereas mammalian cells consist of a 60/40s make-up
   - Chloramphenicol inhibits 50s subunit transpeptidation
   - Macrolides (e.g. erythromycin) prevent translocation
   - Tetracyclines block the binding of tRNA within the 30s subunit
   - Aminoglycosides (e.g. gentamicin) also block binding within the 30s subunit and cause miscoding of the mRNA chain

b) Antibiotic Prophylaxis

- Antimicrobials should be given prior to a procedure likely to result in bacteraemia; plasma levels are therapeutic when exposure to micro-organisms occurs
- Results in smaller systemic effects from the bacteraemia, reducing the possibility of subsequent infection

- Aims to ↓ effects of skin flora being inoculated into the circulation and should be guided by surgical site
- Commonly used in surgical procedures involving implantation of foreign material (i.e. orthopaedics and general surgery)
- Also commonplace in procedures with high probability of bacteraemia (i.e. cystoscopy and other urological procedures)
- Medical prophylaxis is used in people exposed to patients at high risk of transferring infections (e.g. meningococcal meningitis)
- The cornerstone of this principle is the timing of the infusion to coincide with bacterial inoculation. Antibiotics are usually administered at induction:
  - ◆ optimum timing approximately 30 minutes before knife to skin
  - ◆ if antibiotics are administered too early, peak plasma concentration will fall, reducing bacterial penetration; late administration will have a similar effect
- Use of a tourniquet to isolate the surgical site must also be taken into consideration, ensuring drugs are given with adequate time for delivery to the surgical site
- Despite popular surgical belief, prolonged administration of antibiotics (1–2 days postoperatively) has demonstrated no benefit

i) Advantages
  - ↓ incidence of wound infection and improved tissue healing
  - Shorter postoperative recovery period

ii) Disadvantages
  - Risk of allergic reactions ranging from mild to life-threatening, especially to the penicillin-based drugs
  - Repeated exposure can increase the incidence of multi-resistant organism development in the gut
  - Removal of protective colonization (e.g. cephalosporins), resulting in *Clostridium difficile* infection
  - Aminoglycosides can interfere with drug metabolism (e.g. warfarin, NDMBs)
  - Poor evidence base to support use of antibiotic prophylaxis in certain types of surgery
  - Difficulty with timing administration of antimicrobials to have maximal effect
  - Broad-spectrum antibiotics not tailored to likely organism and site of inoculation; usually protocol based

Notes

....

....

....

....

....

....

References

Culver DH, Horan TC, Gaynes RP, *et al.* (1991). Surgical wound infection rates by wound class, operative procedure, and patient risk index. National Nosocomial Infections Surveillance System. *American Journal of Medicine*, **91**: 152S–7S, 1991

Varley AJ, Sule J, Absalom AR. Principles of antibiotic therapy. *Continuing Education in Anaesthesia, Critical Care & Pain*, **9**: 184–8, 2009

Q6 Blood Transfusion

a) **What procedures exist to minimize incorrect transfusion of red blood cells to patients? (5 marks)**

b) **What clinical parameters guide the decision whether to transfuse patients? (4 marks)**

c) **Describe the perioperative alternatives to transfusion of allogeneic blood (11 marks)**

Aims

Both safety and financial issues are covered here. AAGBI publications are a popular source of SAQ and SOE material because of their topical nature so be sure to go through recent 'releases' prior to the examination.

a) Minimization of Incorrect Transfusion

- Confirmation of patient's identity: name, date of birth, hospital number
- Check compatibility of patient's blood group and expiry date
- Ensure blood that is removed from the refrigerator for >30 minutes is used within 4 hours or disposed of
- Accurate records: clinical observations (including temperature during transfusion), timings of transfusion, product identity numbers; to be recorded on a dedicated transfusion care pathway or document, or in the clinical notes
- Ability to trace transfused blood products is a legal requirement (European Blood Directive)

b) Clinical Parameters

- Based on Hb concentration and clinical situation
- Estimate of Hb concentration using ABG, HemoCue®, formal laboratory results
- Transfusion recommended:
  - in symptomatic patients (i.e. tachycardia, hypotension, dizziness, dyspnoea) with clinical or laboratory evidence of anaemia
  - When Hb <7g/dL; deemed essential when Hb <5g/dL in healthy patients
  - When Hb < 8g/dL in asymptomatic patients with cardiorespiratory disease

c) Perioperative Alternatives

i) Preoperative
  - Autologous donation (blood is collected up to 6 weeks preoperatively, stored in the blood refrigerator, and then transfused when required)
  - Optimize red blood cell production (consider iron, folate, erythropoietin, vitamin B_{12} therapy)
  - Optimize clotting function (consider vitamin K or fresh frozen plasma acutely)
  - Stop anticoagulant and antiplatelet drugs perioperatively. NSAIDs are commonly avoided because of antiplatelet action and risk of causing GI bleeds
  - Acute normovolaemic haemodilution (venesection and replacement with crystalloid or colloid, then re-transfused)

ii) Intraoperative
  - Cell salvage (blood is collected via specialized suction devices, filtered and washed, and then transfused back into the patient)
  - Use of regional techniques; evidence to suggest reduced intraoperative blood loss
  - Surgical skill and technical ability
  - Use of biological haemostatic materials (e.g. Kaltostat®, Surgicel®, fibrin glues)
  - Attention to pressure care and positioning: avoid venous obstruction/hypertension
  - Minimizing venous ooze by avoiding high intrathoracic pressures and hypercapnia during ventilation
  - Maintain core body temperature to minimize hypothermia-related coagulopathy
  - Optimization of oxygen delivery: invasive monitoring, fluid therapy, inotropes, increasing FiO_2 in high-risk patients
  - Administration of anti-fibrinolytics, platelet-activating drugs (e.g. tranexamic acid, desmopressin)
  - Use of recombinant factor VIIa
  - Hypotensive anaesthesia—controversial

iii) Postoperative
  - Ongoing treatment in HDU or ICU
  - Invasive monitoring to guide therapy
  - Optimal O_2 delivery to tissues; may require ongoing mechanical ventilation, fluid therapy, and inotropes
  - Analgesia and sedation to avoid sympathetic stress response, agitation, and pain
  - Minimize venesection and ABG samples

Notes

References

AAGBI. *Blood Transfusion and the Anaesthetist. Red Cell Transfusion 2.* London: AAGBI, 2008
Milligan LJ, Bellamy MC. Anaesthesia and critical care of Jehovah's Witnesses. *Continuing Education in Anaesthesia, Critical Care & Pain*, **4**: 35–9, 2004

Q7 Cell Salvage

a) **List the indications for using intraoperative cell salvage (ICS) (4 marks)**

b) **Describe the mechanisms by which blood from the surgical site is collected and processed to produce packed red cells for transfusion (6 marks)**

c) **Discuss the use of ICS in i) obstetric patients (4 marks), ii) patients with malignancy (3 marks), and iii) surgery with bowel contamination (3 marks)**

Aims

Faced with the risks of red cell transfusion, ICS is gradually becoming more commonplace in most hospitals. The scenarios where its use is recommended or clearly contraindicated are becoming more defined, and publications of guidelines regarding its use make it an easy topic to add to the SAQ paper.

a) Indications

- Where major haemorrhage is predicted, i.e. >1000mL or >20% of estimated blood volume
- In patients who present with an ↑ risk of bleeding (e.g. clotting disorders, sepsis)
- In patients with an identified preoperative anaemia
- In patients with unusual blood types or known identified antibodies
- In patients who refuse allogeneic blood donation (e.g. Jehovah's Witnesses). It is important to obtain consent for use of ICS in these patients, as some may also refuse this

b) Mechanisms of ICS

- The surgeon is given a specially adapted dual-lumen suction catheter to use. Blood is collected from the operative site, anticoagulated as it is aspirated via the suction catheter, and delivered to a sterile collection reservoir by vacuum
- Clots and gross debris are removed as blood travels through a 40µm in-line leucodepletion filter into a centrifuge chamber
- Using centrifugation, blood is separated into denser packed red cells, which remain in the centrifuge bowl, and waste products (e.g. white blood cells, platelets, plasma, anticoagulant and fat products), which are forced out into a separate waste line and disposed of
- The packed red cells are washed with a sterile isotonic saline solution and pumped into a separate collecting bag
- Collected packed red cells may be either re-transfused immediately or stored for 6 hours
- Blood-soaked swabs (which account for a large volume of blood loss) may also be washed, and the resulting blood-wash mix placed in the collection reservoir

c) Special Circumstances

i) Obstetric Patients
   - ICS is becoming more popular in obstetric cases with a risk of massive obstetric haemorrhage (e.g. Caesarean section in placental implantation syndromes)
   - Initial fears of risk of amniotic fluid embolism due to reinfusion of fetal substances are unfounded; no reports are described in the literature
   - ICS use in obstetrics is recommended by NICE
   - Be aware of potential rhesus incompatibility, i.e. Rh −ve mother receiving cell-salvaged blood contaminated with Rh +ve fetal blood. Anti-D should be administered
   - Use of double suction set-up recommended: one suction system for blood and ICS and the other for amniotic fluid

ii) Malignancy
- ICS is not recommended by manufacturers for use in malignancy cases because of the risk of reinfusing malignant cells and formation of metastases
- No evidence of malignant recurrence of cancer due to use of ICS in the literature
- Recommended for use in urological malignancy surgery (e.g. radical prostatectomy) by NICE. Advised to minimize suction of blood around the tumour site and use leucodepletion filters to limit malignant cell numbers

iii) Bowel Contamination
- ICS has been relatively contraindicated in the past unless massive haemorrhage was present, although it has been shown that postoperative wound infection rates are unaltered when ICS is required
- Common sense required: remove as much bowel contaminant as possible prior to ICS, use broad-spectrum antibiotics, and increase the volume of wash used during the ICS process

Notes

References

AAGBI. *Blood Transfusion and the Anaesthetist. Intra-operative Cell Salvage.* AAGBI Safety Guideline. London: AAGBI, 2009

NICE. *Intraoperative Red Blood Cell Salvage During Radical Prostatectomy or Radical Cystectomy.* NICE Guidance No. 258, April 2008. Available online at: http://guidance.nice.org.uk/IPG258 (accessed 29 September 2009)

NICE. *Intraoperative Blood Cell Salvage in Obstetrics.* NICE Guidance No. 144, November 2005. Available online at: http://guidance.nice.org.uk/IPG144 (accessed 29 September 2009)

Q8 Creutzfeldt–Jakob disease

a) What processes exist for the decontamination of theatre equipment? (4 marks)

b) Define Creutzfeldt–Jakob disease (6 marks)

c) What important factors are involved in minimizing the risk of intraoperative transmission of Creutzfeldt–Jakob disease? (10 marks)

Aims

Equipment decontamination, another topic disliked by candidates, seems to make regular appearances in FRCA examinations in one guise or another. Do not be caught out!

a) Decontamination Processes

- Cleaning: removal of debris by washing with detergent, rinsing, and drying. Optimizes effectiveness of disinfection and sterilization of equipment
- Disinfection: use of substances such as 2% chlorhexidine in 70% alcohol or sodium hypochlorite kills most bacteria (except endospores and TB), fungi, and viruses. Further disinfection with substances like aldehydes is more effective and may produce sterilization over a longer period of time
- Sterilization: processes such as autoclaving remove all bacteria, viruses, spores, and fungi

b) Creutzfeldt–Jakob disease

- A transmissible spongiform encephalopathy caused by an abnormal infectious prion protein
- Divided into sporadic, hereditary, and acquired cases
- Acquired cases are transmitted by contaminated surgical equipment and tissue transplantation (e.g. cornea or dura mater, immunoglobulins, or human pituitary growth hormone injections)
- Variant form: the prion protein may also be found in the tonsils, appendix, and lymph nodes
- Diagnosis is characterized by a progressive fatal neurological deterioration (e.g. neuropsychiatric disorders, cerebellar symptoms, unusual sensory symptoms ('sticky skin'))
- Diagnosis is made by MRI, electroencephalography, tonsillar biopsy, and CSF sampling

c) Minimizing Intraoperative Transmission

- Standard universal infection control precautions apply
- Use of full aseptic precautions for invasive procedures (e.g. central venous cannulation) including visors and masks to protect the face
- Identification of tissue at increased risk of infectivity (e.g. tonsils, adenoids, posterior eye, brain, spinal cord)
- Communication with haematology and microbiology regarding the management and portering of tissue and blood specimens, and their risk of infectivity
- Equipment that potentially may be in contact with high-risk tissue (e.g. brain or spinal cord) must be either quarantined or destroyed after use (e.g. laryngoscopes and bronchoscopes)
- Airway equipment used for tonsillectomy and/or adenoidectomy should be thrown away postoperatively
- The use of disposable equipment must be encouraged where reliably and economically possible (e.g. laryngoscope blades)
- Re-usable equipment should have tracing protocols in place

- Efforts must be made to reduce the risk of transmission via blood products:
  - minimize the use of blood products intraoperatively
  - leucodepletion of white blood cells
  - obtain the majority of plasma cells from outside the UK

Notes

Reference

AAGBI. *Infection in Anaesthesia 2.* AAGBI Safety Guideline. London: AAGBI, 2008

Q9 Contrast-Induced Nephropathy

a) Define contrast-induced nephropathy (CIN) (2 marks)

b) Outline the pathophysiology of this phenomenon (6 marks)

c) List risk factors for developing CIN (6 marks)

d) Describe factors that may reduce the likelihood of developing CIN (6 marks)

Aims

CME review articles in the major anaesthetic journals provide material for both the written and oral sections of the examination. Anaesthetists are often asked whether it is appropriate to give IV contrast for imaging purposes; we must be aware of the risks involved and the steps taken to reduce the incidence and severity.

a) Definition

- A temporal link between renal function deterioration and administration of IV contrast in the absence of other aetiology
- Absolute ↑ of serum creatinine of 44μmol/L, or relative ↑ of 25% from baseline levels

b) Pathophysiology

- Medullary hypoxia via:
  - prolonged vasoconstriction 2° to adenosine, endothelin, tubuloglomerular feedback, and direct action on vascular smooth muscle
  - altered autoregulation of renal vasculature
- Reperfusion injury via free-radical attack
- Evidence of direct tubular cytotoxicity
- Pre-existing or exacerbated systemic factors contribute towards these processes (see below)

c) Risk Factors

- Elderly
- Premorbid renal dysfunction, including sepsis
- Comorbidities (e.g. diabetes mellitus, congestive heart failure)
- Peri-procedural hypovolaemia
- Peri-procedural anaemia
- Concomitant use of nephrotoxic drugs
- Volume and type of contrast used

d) Prophylaxis

- Identification of patients at risk
- Adequate peri-procedural hydration: crystalloid of choice (e.g. Hartmann's solution or isotonic saline) as a fluid load prior to the procedure
- Avoidance of nephrotoxic drugs (e.g. diuretics, NSAIDs, aminoglycosides)
- Some evidence to suggest:
  - anti-oxidants (e.g. N-acetylcysteine, ascorbic acid): antioxidants used as a free-radical scavenger and renal vasodilatory effect
  - statins: modify endothelial function and inflammatory pathways

Prophylactic haemofiltration in the ICU reduces the incidence and mortality of CIN but is invasive, impractical, expensive, and requires trained staff.

Notes

Reference

Wong GT, Irwin MG. Contrast-induced nephropathy. *British Journal of Anaesthesia*, **99**: 474–83, 2007

Q10 Cervical Spine Trauma

You are asked to provide airway management for a 32-year-old woman involved in a high-speed traffic accident. Her cervical spine is immobilized and her GCS is 6/15.

a) Discuss techniques which may be used to minimize secondary spinal cord injury in this patient whilst securing her airway (10 marks)

b) List the clinical implications of anaesthetising this patient 6 months post C5–6 spinal cord injury (10 marks)

Aims

Secondary spinal cord injury carries high morbidity and mortality. Your answer will need to present an ordered approach to airway management whilst clearly demonstrating an awareness of the chance of pre-existing or subsequent cervical spine trauma and its prevention.

a) Minimization of Secondary Cord Injury

- Airway assessment: difficulty in intubation is common in this cohort:
  - No ability to assess range of movement at the occipito–atlanto-axial junction
  - Mouth opening and jaw slide are impinged by the rigid collar
  - Reduced conscious state further complicates the airway assessment
- A balance must be struck between the need for intubation using a technique with which you are suitably familiar and preventing further cord injury
- A second senior anaesthetist should be involved. Transfer the patient to a familiar environment (i.e. theatre) if stable; a trained anaesthetic assistant should be present
- Ensure that difficult airway equipment is present and checked before embarking on semi-elective difficult airway patients
- If a difficult intubation is predicted in the presence of a full stomach (trauma, pain, opioids), an awake fibreoptic technique may be the safest option. However, in semi-conscious patients ± facial fractures, bleeding, partial obstruction, there is significant risk of failure or complications
- Basic airway manoeuvres cause as much displacement of the cervical spine as direct laryngoscopy. Therefore RSI is the safest option in a patient with predicted relatively easy intubation and poses little additional risk when used with manual in-line stabilization
- Suxamethonium would be acceptable to use at this stage of the spinal cord injury
- Neurological injury is more likely to occur due to ↓ perfusion 2° to hypotension than mechanical displacement. BP monitoring is essential before and after sedation/intubation
- New equipment such as the Glidescope® or Airtraq® may be advantageous by optimizing the view of the laryngeal inlet whilst minimizing cervical spine manipulation

b) Anaesthetic Management of Cord Injury

i) Central Nervous System
  - The patient may be hypertonic and hyper-reflexic with a significant risk of autonomic dysreflexia to nociceptive and proprioceptive stimulation below the level of the lesion
  - Difficult assessment of patient if associated traumatic brain injury or altered affect
  - Assessment of postoperative pain is challenging

ii) Airway
  - Potential for difficult intubation (see above); may have had cervical spinal surgery (e.g. fixation (limited neck movement))

- Suxamethonium is avoided because of the risk of arrhythmias or cardiac arrest 2° to hyperkalaemia

iii) Respiratory
- ↓ spirometry values (e.g. functional residual capacity, vital capacity)
- Poor cough and secretion clearance: ↑ risk for aspiration and postoperative chest infection
- Phrenic nerve function impairment if lesion at C4: assessed by flow volume loops and video fluoroscopy. Ventilation often better supine because of cephalic diaphragm displacement
- ↑ postoperative respiratory support may be required

iv) Cardiovascular
- Postural hypotension is common
- Consequences of autonomic dysreflexia (i.e. bradycardia, hypertension) can cause acute MI, heart failure, and pulmonary oedema. Treat with sublingual GTN initially
- Exaggerated response to hypotension following blood loss or regional blocks

v) Gastrointestinal
- Consider modified RSI: ↑ risk of aspiration on induction 2° to delayed gastric emptying

vi) Genitourinary
- ↑ incidence of UTI due to permanent in-dwelling catheters or poor bladder emptying leads to ↑ risk of sepsis and presence of stones, especially following instrumentation
- Possibility of renal failure subsequent to repeated infections

vii) Other
- ↑ incidence of postoperative DVT: consider thromboprophylactic requirements
- Osteoporosis and pathological fractures occur: care with transfer and handling of patient
- Difficulty in positioning patients with hypertonic contractures
- Deranged thermoregulation and shivering: ensure adequate temperature control
- Chronic malnutrition is common in this cohort

Notes

....

....

....

....

....

....

....

....

....

....

Q11 Day Surgery

a) **List the patient selection criteria for day surgery (6 marks)**

b) **What are the important organizational (7 marks) and anaesthetic (7 marks) considerations governing the perioperative care of day surgery**

Aims

With financial constraints tightening the NHS, there is more pressure to increase day surgery and free up hospital beds. This is topical and extremely relevant.

a) Criteria

i) Medical
- Normally fit and well, *or* well-controlled chronic disease (i.e. diabetes, hypertension)
- Patients should be able to understand the benefits and risks of the procedure, including postoperative care. This extends to any immediate carers

NB: Obesity is not an absolute contraindication to day surgery, depending on facilities, expertise, etc.

ii) Social
- Patients must be able to attend preoperative assessment clinics
- There must be a responsible adult to transport the patient home and oversee the first 24 hours of postoperative care
- The patient should have access to a telephone for advice and emergencies
- The patient's accommodation should be suitable for postoperative care, i.e. adequate heating, hot water, and toilet facilities

b) Considerations

i) Organizational
- There should be a designated purpose-built hospital area or ward for the day surgery unit
- A lead senior clinician (ideally a consultant anaesthetist with a specialist interest in day surgery) is responsible for developing protocols, guidelines, clinical governance, and training
- A senior nurse is in charge of the day-to-day running of the unit. There is direct liaison with the unit's lead clinician. They will also be responsible for clinical governance, rotas, staffing, and day surgery training
- Representation at trust board level is desirable
- Dedicated suitably skilled clerical staff should be available
- If day-case paediatric surgery is offered, facilities to provide a service to standards expected of a paediatric surgical ward is mandatory (may require separate unit)
- There must be adequate resources for catering facilities
- List order: ideally day-case patients should be at the beginning, allowing for adequate recovery time throughout the day prior to discharge home
- There must be clear and concise discharge criteria guidelines for all day surgery patients, usually based on either clinical parameters or scoring systems
- A copy of the discharge summary should be provided for the patient and GP, which should also be filed in the hospital notes

- Appropriate verbal and written advice for postoperative care regarding driving, cooking, drinking alcohol, contact numbers, and follow-up clinics must be given to patients at discharge

ii) Anaesthetic
  - Compulsory preoperative assessment and optimization of chronic conditions is imperative to a successful clinical outcome for day surgery, i.e. uneventful perioperative period with same-day discharge home
  - Analgesia: aim for pain-free postoperative period by using a combination of analgesics, i.e. paracetamol, NSAIDs (if not contraindicated), weak to moderate opioids (e.g. tramadol, codeine phosphate), and short-acting opioids (e.g. fentanyl, alfentanil)
  - Consider use of regional techniques if possible and appropriate: separate criteria for discharge may be required (e.g. minimal or no opiate adjunct, lower volume of LA, ability to pass urine)
  - Postoperative nausea and vomiting: identification of high-risk patients and suitable modification of anaesthetic techniques (e.g. total IV anaesthesia, multi-modal anti-emetic prophylaxis, IV fluid therapy)
  - Evidence shows that standard anaesthesia and analgesia protocols for certain operations (e.g. laparoscopic cholecystectomy) minimizes morbidity and allows successful same-day discharge
  - Guidelines for prescription of discharge medication, specifically analgesia (multimodal as above)

Notes

Reference

AAGBI. *Day Surgery* (revised). London: AAGBI, 2005

Q12 Electroconvulsive Therapy

You are asked to anaesthetise patients for an electroconvulsive therapy list at a small local district general hospital.

a) List the problems associated with this type of list (5 marks)

b) Describe the physiological changes that occur during ECT treatment (3 marks)

c) Outline a suitable anaesthetic technique for this list (12 marks)

Aims

This SAQ combines a procedure that many will not have performed, with several service issues such as distant-site anaesthesia and patients with potentially significant comorbidities and pharmacological drug interactions. The examiners will want to see how the candidate approaches dealing with difficult patients in a remote site. This SAQ is all about awareness of the situation. Be safe!

a) Problems

- Anaesthesia at a remote isolated site
- Equipment: may be old, neglected, not serviced or checked, unfamiliar
- Drugs: limited range, may be out of date
- Resuscitation: limited equipment, access, or support
- Staff: limited experience or anaesthetic knowledge
- Patients: challenging (!), poor historians, polypharmacy with potential for anaesthetic drug interactions (e.g. monoamine oxidase inhibitors)

b) Physiological Changes

- Initially parasympathetic stimulation: bradycardia and hypotension for 10–20 seconds
- Then extended sympathetic surge: tachycardia, arrhythmias, hypertension
- ↑ ICP, IOP, cerebral blood flow, intragastric pressure, secretions

c) Anaesthetic Technique

- Standard anaesthetic preoperative assessment but with the above challenges
- Probably previous ECT: check anaesthetic charts for technique or problems
- Ensure no contraindications (e.g. recent MI or CVA, intracranial pathology (aneurysm, tumour), glaucoma, or long-bone fractures)
- Consider anti-sialogogue premedication (e.g. glycopyrrolate 200mcg IV)
- Ensure thorough checking of anaesthetic equipment and drugs, including adequate airway back-up facilities
- Ensure skilled experienced assistant available
- IV induction (e.g. propofol)
- Seizure modification: suxamethonium 0.5–1mg/kg to prevent injury
- Maintain airway with face mask ± oropharyngeal airway
- Insert bite block to protect tongue, teeth, and oral mucosa
- Ventilate with 100% O_2 until spontaneous respiration returns
- Further doses of IV induction agent may be required if multiple seizures are induced
- Opiates or β-blockers may be used to obtund sympathetic surges
- Benzodiazepines may be used if seizures are prolonged
- Postoperative simple analgesia for headaches or muscular pain

- If complications (e.g. cardiac ischaemia or bone fractures) suspected:
  - ABC approach and institute necessary urgent treatment where possible
  - involve relevant medical or surgical specialties for further care

Notes

Reference

O'Donnell A. Anaesthesia for electroconvulsive therapy (ECT). In: Allman KG, Wilson I, eds, *Oxford Handbook of Anaesthesia* (2nd edn). Oxford University Press, 2006; 280–1

Q13 Epidural Abscess

You are called to review the epidural site of a 69-year-old man 3 days post anterior resection. He is pyrexial and has developed acute back pain.

a) What are the risk factors for developing an epidural abscess? (6 marks)

b) List examinations and investigations which may confirm your diagnosis (7 marks)

c) Outline the management of this patient (7 marks)

Aims

We cannot stress strongly enough the need to take signs and symptoms of an epidural abscess seriously and act appropriately with urgent imaging for diagnosis. Being able to stratify risk factors rapidly, and examine and investigate a patient, will expedite prompt management and potentially improve outcome.

a) Risk Factors

- Immunocompromised patients (e.g. steroid use, diabetes mellitus, HIV, cancer, chemo- or radiotherapy, alcohol or IV drug abuse, pregnancy)
- Primary infection (e.g. soft tissue, presence of an intravenous cannula) with secondary spread to the spinal column (exacerbated in the immunocompromised, as above)
- Central neuraxial block: repeated attempts, poor aseptic technique, minor coagulopathy (haematoma = ideal bacterial growth medium), catheter *in situ* for >4 days, catheter dressing promoting moist skin, break in integrity of epidural drug delivery system
- Other breaches of spinal column integrity (e.g. surgery, instrumentation, trauma, vertebral collapse secondary to osteoarthritis or osteoporosis)

b) Investigations

i) Examination
- Inspection of epidural catheter insertion site: evidence of subcutaneous infection raises suspicion
- Full neurological examination looking for warning signs (e.g. motor or sensory deficit, diminished or absent reflexes, incontinence, meningism)

ii) Investigations
- Blood tests: raised inflammatory markers (WCC, CRP) are non-specific and there may be other confounding factors. ESR is persistently raised (>30mm/hour) and is more specific
- Cultures:
    - need to identify any potential primary infection site (e.g. CXR, urine MC&S, wound swabs)
    - common bacterial organisms include: *Staphylococcus aureus*, streptococci, and various Gram −ve bacilli (e.g. *Escherichia coli*, proteus, and pseudomonas species)
    - less common: mycobacterial, fungal, and parasitic abscesses
- Radiology:
    - spine radiographs: only diagnostic in a minority of patients
    - myelography: invasive and potential spread of infection
    - CT spine: previously the gold standard, but now replaced by MRI
    - whole-spine MRI with gadolinium = *investigation of choice*

c) Management

- Immediate removal of epidural catheter. Send catheter tip for culture
- Prolonged IV antibiotic therapy: guided by microbiology department and adjusted according to culture results. Initially IV for 3–4 weeks; then converted to oral for a further 6–8 weeks
- Regular clinical monitoring of temperature, epidural catheter entry site, functional neurology, and inflammatory markers to guide therapy

i) Non-surgical
  - Criteria: minor neurology, already on IV antibiotics, poor surgical candidate because of comorbidities, abscess so large that surgery would destroy the spinal structure
  - CT-guided percutaneous drainage of abscess more rarely

ii) Surgical
  - Early open surgical decompression of abscess if:
    - rapid-onset neurological deterioration
    - extensive or loculated appearance
    - failed medical therapy
  - During surgery: debridement, pus swabs for MC&S and AAFB, tissue histology

Notes

References

Simpson KH, Said Al-Makadma Y. Epidural drug delivery and spinal infection. *Continuing Education in Anaesthesia, Critical Care & Pain*, **7**: 112–15, 2007

Grewal S, Hocking G, Wildsmith JA. Epidural abscesses. *British Journal of Anaesthesia*, **96**: 292–302, 2006

Q14 **Ethics 1**

You are anaesthetising a 56-year-old man, in a UK hospital, who has given consent for an arthroscopic subacromial decompression of his left shoulder. During the procedure, the surgeon announces that he has identified a previously undiagnosed rotator cuff tear and proposes to repair it.

a) Is it lawful for the surgeon to proceed and repair the torn rotator cuff? (3 marks)

b) Who takes responsibility for the decision? (3 marks)

During the procedure, the patient shows signs of a myocardial infarction. An urgent cardiological opinion is sought, and the cardiologist wants to proceed to angioplasty and coronary stent insertion prior to waking the patient.

c) Is it lawful for the cardiologist to proceed to angioplasty and who takes responsibility for this decision? (3 marks)

d) What is the difference between the two situations? (11 marks)

Aims

An entirely plausible scenario exploring the complex area of consent, this question is something of a minefield in the SAQ, made more topical following the Mental Capacity Act 2005 (see Explanatory Notes). It is easy to get bogged down trying to present a balanced argument. Being able to differentiate the two situations clearly using correct terminology will transform this question into one that is much easier to answer.

a) Should the Surgeon Proceed?
- No: a rotator cuff repair is not lawful
- The surgeon will be assaulting the patient as there is no consent for a rotator cuff repair

b) Responsibility
- Shared between surgeon and anaesthetist
- Anaesthetists will be expected to refuse to permit procedures for which no consent has been obtained and there is no other justification for proceeding

c) Angioplasty
- Yes: the angioplasty and insertion of stents is lawful
- Responsibility is shared between cardiologist and anaesthetist

d) Situational Differences
- The difference between the two situations is that the MI is an immediate threat to life
- Treatment of the MI may continue on the basis of the patient's 'best interests'
- Waking the patient prior to insertion of stents may result in the patient dying before consent can be obtained
- There is no similar justification for performing a rotator cuff repair.
- The patient's life is not in any immediate danger
- A full discussion of the pros and cons of a repair can proceed after completion of the decompression

Explanatory Notes

The Mental Capacity Act 2005 applies to English and Welsh jurisdictions. Similar principles apply in Scotland and Northern Ireland. In Scotland the law is bound by the Adults with Incapacity (Scotland) Act 2001. In Northern Ireland, there is no statute law at present, but common law supports a similar situation to the answer provided. Further reading for a complete explanation is advised for practitioners in Scotland and Northern Ireland.

Notes

References

AAGBI. *Consent for Anaesthesia* (revised). London: AAGBI, 2006

Danbury CM, Newdick C, Lawson A, Waldmann CS (eds). *Law and Ethics in Intensive Care.* Oxford University Press, 2010

Mason JK, Laurie GT. *Mason and McCall Smith's Law and Medical Ethics.* Oxford University Press, 2010

Q15 **Ethics 2**

In England, a 39-year-old woman is admitted to the neurointensive care unit with a closed head injury following a motor vehicle accident. After discussion with the neurosurgeons, no surgical intervention is indicated at present, and it has been decided to keep this woman sedated and ventilated. Her husband arrives and states that pre-accident she had been terrified of living with such a brain injury. He insists that treatment be withdrawn, allowing her to die.

a) Should his demands be followed? Explain how you come to your conclusion (7 marks)

Treatment is not withdrawn. The husband returns with a document signed by his wife purporting to give him Lasting Power of Attorney (LPA). He states that this gives him the legal power to refuse treatment on behalf of his wife. He demands that treatment is withdrawn.

b) Does an LPA give the Attorney the right to refuse treatment? (2 marks)

c) Has the husband provided sufficient information to prove that he has an LPA? (3 marks)

d) Does the fact that he appears to have a signed LPA mean that his demands should be followed? Justify your answer (8 marks)

Aims

This is a difficult clinical scenario and not an easy SAQ. Although the initial answer seems obvious, justifying it becomes trickier. Being able to demonstrate a familiarity with the legal framework that operates in this area is required not just for examination answers but also for clinical practice.

a) Demands

- No, his demands should not be followed without a full discussion and determination of the patient's 'best interests'
- The husband's views are evidence of the patient's wishes, but are not in themselves determinative
- Other family members may provide different views of the woman's wishes
- Even then, at this early stage it is impossible to determine whether she will have any lasting significant brain injury

b) Lasting Power of Attorney

- Yes, an LPA which covers medical treatment decisions and specifies life and death decision-making, gives the Attorney the right to refuse treatment

c) Information

- No, the husband will need to register the LPA with the Court of Protection after his wife has lost capacity to consent. This takes time
- When the LPA is granted, the Court will provide appropriate documentation to the husband to prove his position

d) Demands

If there is a dispute between clinicians and the Attorney (appointed by an LPA), and it is the belief of the clinicians that the Attorney is not acting in the 'best interests' of the patient, then you *must* return to the Court to seek a review

- The Court of Protection can:
  - ◆ make a decision itself
  - ◆ confirm the Attorney's decision
  - ◆ remove the Attorney and appoint a Deputy to make further decisions on behalf of the Court of Protection

Explanatory Notes

The Mental Capacity Act 2005 applies to English and Welsh jurisdictions. Similar principles apply in Scotland and Northern Ireland. In Scotland the law is bound by the Adults with Incapacity (Scotland) Act 2001. In Northern Ireland, there is no statute law at present, but common law supports a similar situation to the answer provided. Further reading for a complete explanation is advised for practitioners in Scotland and Northern Ireland.

Notes

References

AAGBI. *Consent for Anaesthesia* (revised). London: AAGBI, 2006

Danbury CM, Newdick C, Lawson A, Waldmann CS, eds. *Law and Ethics in Intensive Care.* Oxford University Press, 2010

Mental Capacity Act 2005. Available online at: http://www.dca.gov.uk/menincap/mca-act-easyread. pdf (accessed May 2010)

Q16 Evoked Potentials

a) Draw a labelled diagram of i) an action potential in a peripheral axon, ii) a cardiac action potential (5 marks)

b) Describe how membrane permeability to key ions renders a cell excitable (9 marks)

c) Discuss the clinical applications of evoked potentials in anaesthesia and intensive care (6 marks)

Aims

The key to diagrams being successful in the examination is to ensure that they are clear, simple, and well labelled. Practice before the examination makes them easier to reproduce under time constraints and is highly recommended. The use of evoked potentials in clinical practice at first seems vague, but closer inspection reveals that they are commonly used.

a) Labelled Diagrams

i) Peripheral Axon

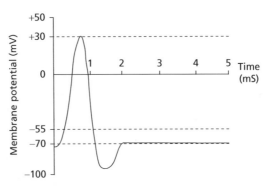

Figure 1. Peripheral axon

ii) Cardiac Action Potential

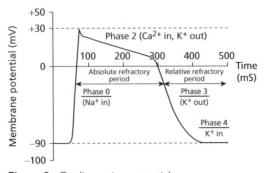

Figure 2. Cardiac action potential

b) Membrane Permeability

- All mammalian cells are enclosed by a phospholipid bilayer: the cell membrane
- A physicochemical gradient is established, allowing selective ion permeability
- This potential is responsible for allowing a cell to be termed excitable
- The membrane is relatively impermeable to most cations except K^+
- The intracellular concentration of K^+ is higher (150mM) than the extracellular concentration (5mM)
- K^+ leaks out of the cell down its concentration gradient; this is terminated by the electrical gradient that develops due to impermeability of the membrane to other ions
- Resting membrane potential (RMP): where the chemical gradient of K^+ *out* of the cell equals the electrical gradient pulling K^+ *into* the cell (usually around −70mV)
- The main extracellular anion is Cl^-; a similar equilibrium is established by balancing its electrochemical gradient
- The relative impermeability of the membrane to Na^+ helps to maintain its electrochemical gradient *into* the cell
- However, small amounts of Na^+ leak intracellularly; the $3Na^+/2K^+/ATPase$ pump is responsible for neutralizing this effect
- Active pumping of Na^+ *out* of the cell allows the Na^+ gradient to be maintained
- Without this pump, the RMP would gradually disappear and cells would be rendered unexcitable
- Similar mechanisms exist for other ions, for example Ca^{2+} (maintained at low concentrations by membrane expulsion of the ion, whilst at higher concentrations Ca^{2+} is exchanged for Na^+ ions which are subsequently cleared via the $Na^+/K^+/ATPase$ pump)
- The membrane potential is the result of the equilibrium of multiple ions, and the individual charge can be calculated using the Nernst equation
- The Goldmann–Hodgkin–Katz equation aims to combine the effect of multiple ions to generate the overall RMP
- For a cell to be termed excitable, a feature is present in the membrane which, following an appropriate trigger, confers a change in membrane permeability followed by a flux of cations intracellularly (predominantly Na^+)
- Ion channels or intracellular messenger systems are usually responsible. A process to restore the resting potential must also be in place in order to reset the mechanics for subsequent stimuli

c) Evoked Potentials in Anaesthesia and the ICU

i) Anaesthesia
- Depth of anaesthesia (auditory evoked potentials (AEPs) superior to others) Anaesthetic agents decrease the amplitude and increase the latency of the early and mid-cortical AEPs in a dose-dependent, but agent-independent, manner. The early and late responses are unaffected by anaesthetic agents
- Degree of muscle paralysis with peripheral nerve stimulator
- Neurosurgery: to confirm the integrity of neural pathways during tissue dissection (e.g. spinal surgery or acoustic neuroma)
- During carotid endarterectomy under GA, more sensitive to subtle ischaemic changes than EEG monitoring. However, the response of the system is slower
- Visual evoked potentials: test integrity of visual pathways during neurosurgery around visual pathway and cortex
- Some research has shown somatosensory evoked potentials to be a more sensitive method of assessing epidural level of blockade

ii) ICU
- As a prognostic aid in traumatic brain injury with an intact brainstem. Poor prognosis associated with anoxic brain injury and bilaterally absent evoked potentials
- Integrity of nerve pathways in investigating paralysed limbs, i.e. traumatic plexopathy
- Diagnosis of neuropathy and myopathy, and the ability to distinguish between them
- Monitoring of neuromuscular blocking levels in patients on infusions of muscle relaxants

Notes

References

Duffy CM, Manninen PH, Chan A, Kearns CF (1997). Comparison of cerebral oximeter and evoked potential monitoring in carotid endarterectomy. *Canadian Journal of Anaesthesia*, **44**: 1077–81

Gajraj RJ, Doi M, Mantzaridis H, Kenny GN (1999). Comparison of bispectral EEG analysis and auditory evoked potentials for monitoring depth of anaesthesia during propofol anaesthesia. *British Journal of Anaesthesia*, **82**: 672–8

Zaric, D., S. Hallgren, Leissner L, *et al.* (1996). Evaluation of epidural sensory block by thermal stimulation, laser stimulation, and recording of somatosensory evoked potentials. *Regional Anesthesia*, **21**: 124–38

http://emedicine.medscape.com/article/1137451-overview (accessed 25 March 2010)

Q17 Extubation

a) **Which groups of patient are at high risk of problems during extubation? (8 marks)**

b) **List potential causes of laryngospasm post-extubation (5 marks)**

c) **Outline a strategy for managing laryngospasm (7 marks)**

Aims

A great deal of emphasis is placed on teaching intubation and relatively little on supervised extubation. The ability to manage post-extubation laryngospasm is core knowledge and should be answered as such. No margins for error here in safety!

a) High-Risk Patients

i) Patient Factors
   - Obesity, OSA
   - Severe cardiorespiratory disease
   - Reflux
   - Congenital or acquired airway pathology (e.g. burns, radiotherapy, tumour, trauma)
   - Bony or soft tissue abnormalities (e.g. craniofacial, implants, cervical spine fixation)

ii) Anaesthetic Factors
   - Repeated intubation attempts
   - Extubation attempt in lighter planes of anaesthesia

iii) Surgical Factors
   - Airway surgery (e.g. oedema, bleeding, tracheomalacia, swelling, laryngeal damage)
   - Neck, thyroid, or dental surgery (e.g. abscess drainage, oedema, altered anatomy, haematoma, recurrent laryngeal nerve damage)
   - Limited or ↓ airway access (e.g. wiring, fixation, guardian sutures)
   - Posterior fossa surgery
   - Prolonged surgery in the Trendelenberg position

b) Causes of Laryngospasm

- Presence of blood or secretions in posterior pharynx
- Excessive stimulation or extubation during light planes of anaesthesia
- Airway obstruction (e.g. secondary to oedema, pharyngeal soft tissue collapse)
- Airway irritability (e.g. smokers, URTI)
- Regurgitation and aspiration of stomach contents
- Pain
- Others (e.g. vagal, trigeminal, splanchnic, phrenic nerve stimulation)

c) Stepwise Management of Laryngospasm

- ABC approach and call for help
- Primary aim is oxygenation: give 100% O_2
- Suction airway to remove any secretions / blood
- Oro- or nasopharyngeal airway with jaw thrust
- Apply CPAP with a Mapleson C circuit
- Consider Larson's manoeuvre: combined jaw thrust and direct medial finger-tip pressure posterior to the temporomandibular joint

- Administer IV propofol bolus (usually approximately 20% of the induction dose)
- Administer IV suxamethonium 0.5–1mg/kg (don't forget additional atropine 20mcg/kg in paediatric patients)
- Intubate and ventilate
- Cricothyroidotomy if failure to oxygenate via standard airway devices

Notes

References

Dravid R, Lee G. Extubation and re-intubation strategy. In: Popat M, ed. *Difficult Airway Management*. Oxford University Press, 2009; 131–44

Karmarkar S, Varshney S. Tracheal extubation. *Continuing Education in Anaesthesia, Critical Care & Pain*, **8**: 2008, 214–19

Q18 **Hypotensive Anaesthesia**

You are asked to anaesthetise a 24-year-old woman for middle-ear surgery. The surgeon has requested that you keep the blood pressure low for surgery.

a) Discuss techniques used to provide hypotensive anaesthesia (12 marks)

b) List potential contraindications for this technique (8 marks)

Aims

Successful blood pressure control can make for a shorter easier operation and a happier surgeon! A structured approach looking at the component of blood pressure calculation allows you to identify different areas available for manipulation, whilst not forgetting important complementary non-pharmacological techniques.

a) Hypotensive Techniques

i) Pre-induction
   - Avoid anticholinergic drying agents that may precipitate tachycardia
   - Premedication (e.g. benzodiazepines/opiates): analgesia, anxiolysis, and sedation

ii) Induction
   - Smooth induction in calm environment
   - Only attempt procedures in a deep plane of anaesthesia
   - Avoid etomidate or ketamine for induction
   - Avoid pancuronium for muscle relaxation (precipitates tachycardia)
   - LA spraying of cords at induction to prevent coughing on emergence
   - If appropriate, use an LMA (avoids pressor response to laryngoscopy)

iii) Maintenance
   - Volatile agents may produce hypotension (isoflurane has a direct vessel vasodilator effect)
   - Consider TCI remifentanil and propofol (for titration of blood pressure)
   - IPPV for optimal $PaCO_2$ levels, thereby $\downarrow$ sympathetic tone
   - $\uparrow$ PEEP can be used to $\downarrow$ preload but may precipitate venous hypertension
   - Positioning:
     - elevation of the operative field helps to $\downarrow$ venous bleeding
     - Reverse Trendelenberg positioning to $\downarrow$ right atrial pressure and cardiac output
   - Avoid central and peripheral venous obstruction by keeping the head and limbs unobstructed and without tension

iv) Drugs
   - Classified according to (MAP = CO × SVR)

   CO
   - Short-acting β-blockers (e.g. esmolol or metoprolol) provide negative inotropy whilst preventing compensatory tachycardia

   SVR
   - $\downarrow$ vascular smooth muscle leads to $\downarrow$ BP without reducing cardiac output
   - Direct blockade of the α_1-adrenoceptor: $\downarrow$ arteriole muscular resting tone.
     - Phentolamine: short-acting non-selective α-blocker
     - Prazosin: α_1-blocker but slow in onset

- Clonidine: centrally acting selective α agonist (1:200 α_1:α_2). Initially, $\uparrow$ BP following peripheral α_2 stimulation, then $\downarrow$ BP via noradrenaline inhibition. Analgesic and anxiolytic actions aid its effects
    - Labetalol: α- and β-adrenoceptor blockade (1:7)
- Nitric oxide donors: direct vascular smooth muscle dilatation
    - SNP promotes arterial vasodilation
    - GTN: $\uparrow$ venous capacity by $\uparrow$venous compliance and $\downarrow$ right atrial pressure
- Hydralazine: direct-acting vasodilator; onset time 15 minutes. Cleared in an hour by fast acetylators; precipitates SLE-like crisis in slow acetylators
- Calcium-channel blockers (e.g. nifedipine): vasodilator class of Ca^{2+} anatagonist that dilate vessels and prevent tachycardia
- Sympathetic chain blockade: IV trimetaphan 20–50mcg/kg/min
    - Weak α-blocking actions and direct vasodilator activity. Difficult to titrate

b) Contraindications

i) Cardiovascular Disease
- Any disease state where decreased perfusion may compromise organ function (e.g. cerebrovascular disease, ischaemic heart disease, severe peripheral vascular disease)
- Severe anaemia coupled with reduced CO may precipitate tissue hypoperfusion
- Untreated hypertension:
    - labile blood pressure with unpredictable responses and poor control
    - difficult to predict where lower limits of autoregulation zones lie for core viscera

ii) Respiratory Disease
- Vasodilators abolish hypoxic vasoconstriction
- May $\uparrow$ physiological dead space, FRC, and V/Q mismatch

iii) Other
- Diabetes: sympathetic blockade $\uparrow$ chance of hypoglycaemia
- Pregnancy: placental blood flow is perfusion dependent
- Renal: may precipitate further deterioration in renal function

Notes

Q19 Infection Control

a) Who is responsible for minimizing cross-infection between patients in an operating theatre environment (3 marks)

b) What are the important factors in optimal hand hygiene (5 marks) and the wearing of gloves (5 marks) in the theatre environment?

c) Outline further standard safety procedures that minimize infection transmission in the operating theatre (7 marks)

Aims

This is a hot topic at the moment and has appeared recently in the SAQ paper. It is likely to continue in some form or another, so it is well worth reading about.

a) Responsible Persons

- Trust chief executives
- Trust infection control teams
- Named anaesthetic consultant in department
- Microbiology: to provide advice on decontamination and sterilization
- Occupational health department
- All healthcare workers in contact with the operating theatre

b) Hand Hygiene

i) Optimal Hand Hygiene
   - Hand hygiene is the personal responsibility of *all* theatre staff (current evidence suggests that good hand hygiene is linked with decreased rates of healthcare-associated infections)
   - Regular clinical governance to identify strengths and weaknesses in perioperative infection control
   - Hand decontamination with liquid soap and water prior to every direct patient contact, or if visibly soiled hands
   - If no soiling, use antibacterial hand gel between patient contact (alcohol gel is ineffective against *Clostridium difficile* infection)
   - 'Bare below the elbows' policy, i.e. wristwatches and jewellery removed for entire clinical shift
   - Cuts, abrasions, and skin breaks must be covered with waterproof dressings
   - Known dermatological conditions (e.g. psoriasis) may require occupational health advice or input

ii) Gloves
   - Non-latex gloves must be available for healthcare workers with latex allergy or sensitivity
   - Gloves are single-use items and are put on prior to, and removed directly after, all patient contact
   - Non-sterile gloves should be worn where there may be contact with bodily secretions or mucous membranes, or for non-invasive procedures
   - Sterile gloves must be worn for all invasive procedures
   - Gloves are disposed of as clinical waste in the correct bins

- It is important to avoid touching everyday objects such as computers, telephones, pens, and food with gloves on
- Hands must be decontaminated with liquid soap and water after wearing gloves

c) **Further Safety Procedures**

- Suitable theatre garments (e.g. scrub suits, theatre gowns, disposable theatre caps, and clogs or overshoe covers) must be available for theatre workers
- Provision of face masks is advised as part of an aseptic technique for invasive procedures (e.g. central neuraxial blockade or central venous line insertion). A face guard should also be provided where risk of splash from bodily fluids or secretions is high
- Sharps disposal
  - Adequate disposal containers complying with BS7320: 1990 'Specification for sharps'. Must also follow disposal/incineration protocols
  - Minimal handling of sharps: non-transferrable between clinicians
  - Avoidance of re-sheathing needles
- Theatre list order: infected patients must be easily identifiable on the list so that provisions can be made. Infected patients are commonly put last on the list to minimize transmission to other patients. The theatre is cleaned thoroughly before and after infected cases
- Both infected and non-infected theatre laundry must be disposed of appropriately
- Guidelines to advise the safe preparation and administration of drugs by clinical and non-clinical theatre workers should be adhered to.
  - Single-patient use for needles/syringes (initially stored as sterile in packaging)
  - Single-drug ampoules not shared with multiple patients, and discarded in a suitable sharps containers
  - Infusion preparation: ideally as sterile as possible, avoiding breaks in the system. 'Scrub the hub': use of 2% chlorhexidine gluconate in 70% alcohol to clean IV Luer ports prior to attachment of infusions (avoid three-way taps)

Notes

....

....

....

....

....

....

....

....

....

....

Reference

AAGBI. *Infection in Anaesthesia 2.* AAGBI Safety Guideline. London: AAGBI, 2008

Q20 Intraocular Pressure

You are asked to anaesthetise a 73-year-old woman for corneal grafting under general anaesthesia. She has no other past medical history.

a) List factors which may affect intraocular pressure perioperatively (11 marks)

b) What anaesthetic techniques may be employed to minimize a rise in intraocular pressure? (9 marks)

Aims

The anaesthetic effect on baseline physiology is a common theme for SAQs and you should be able to list how your actions will impact on patients. The obvious reciprocal of this is how we employ techniques to manipulate the physiological response, both pharmacological and non-pharmacological.

a) Factors Affecting Intraocular Pressure

i) External Factors (extraocular compression)
- Anaesthetic equipment e.g. masks
- Surgical equipment e.g. Honan balloon, retractors, surgical hand
- Block complications e.g. ↑ volume of LA, haematoma
- Tumours
- ↑ tone of extrinsic eye muscles e.g. 2° to fasciculations (suxamethonium)

ii) Internal Factors (due to volume of globe contents)
- Aqueous humour volume
- Vitreous humour volume (↑ by haemorrhage)
- Choroid volume (2° to blood volume) depends on:
  - arterial pressure: ↓ volume when SBP < 90mmHg
  - venous pressure: ↑ when venous drainage from head is impaired or on coughing, straining, or laryngoscopy
  - ↑ IOP due to hypercapnia, hypoxaemia
- Presence of foreign body (e.g. sulphur hexafluoride, carbon octafluoride bubble)
- Tumours

iii) Drugs
- All IV anaesthetic induction agents ↓ IOP (except ketamine)
- All anaesthetic volatile agents ↓ IOP moderately
- Suxamethonium ↑ IOP by up to 50%
- N_2O will ↑ IOP if sulphur hexafluoride or carbon octafluoride is used
- Acetazolamide (inhibits carbonic anhydrase) ↓ aqueous humour production
- Mannitol reduces vitreous humour contents by water removal

b) Anaesthetic Techniques
- Careful mask ventilation to avoid globe compression
- Ensure adequate depth of anaesthesia during airway placement to avoid coughing or straining
- LMA, if appropriate, avoids laryngoscopy pressor response
- If intubation is necessary, consider lidocaine spray to vocal cords, opiate, short-acting β-blockers (if not contraindicated) to obtund the pressor response to laryngoscopy

- Consider IV maintenance (e.g. TCI propofol ± remifentanil for smooth intraoperative course and emergence. NDMBs intraoperatively as required
- Aim to minimize venous congestion:
  - Maintain normal $EtCO_2$ levels with IPPV
  - Tape airway securely rather than tying
  - Neutral neck position
  - 15–20° reverse Trendelenberg position on operating table
- IV anti-emetics to prevent postoperative nausea/vomiting
- Avoid surges in BP: adequate anaesthesia, analgesia, muscle relaxation
- Avoid N_2O if sulphur hexafluoride or carbon octafluoride used: O_2 and air instead

Notes

Q21 Local Anaesthetic Toxicity

You have inserted an interpleural catheter into a 54-year-old man with rib fractures following a road traffic accident. After injection of 10ml of 0.375% bupivacaine, the man becomes unresponsive.

a) What are the potential causes of collapse in this man? (2 marks)

b) What signs may lead to a diagnosis of local anaesthetic toxicity? (4 marks)

c) Outline your immediate management of local anaesthetic toxicity. (14 marks)

Aims

This is another SAQ that has recently appeared in the examination. Like anaphylaxis, all doses should be stated accurately and the priorities of treatment established, i.e. ABC. Recent modification of the treatment algorithm should be committed to memory for both clinical practice and the examination.

a) Causes of Collapse

- Local anaesthetic toxicity
- Cardiac: arrest, arrhythmia, CVA, postural hypotension
- Respiratory: hypoxia, hypercarbia, pulmonary embolism, tension pneumothorax
- Endocrine: hypoglycaemia, Addisonian crisis, hypothyroidism
- Other: vasovagal, drugs (e.g. opiates, sedatives), hypovolaemia secondary to bleeding from trauma

b) Signs

- Altered mental state, agitation, loss of consciousness ± generalized tonic–clonic seizures
- Cardiac arrhythmias (e.g. VF, VT, asystole, bradycardia, heart blocks)

c) Management

i) Immediate
  - Stop injecting local anaesthetic
  - Call for help
  - Secure the airway, via endotracheal intubation if appropriate
  - Establish controlled ventilation with 100% oxygen
  - Confirm IV access and manage seizures with standard hypnotics or benzodiazepines (e.g. propofol, thiopentone, diazepam, midazolam)
  - Attach cardiac monitor to assess underlying rhythm
  - Commence CPR if appropriate and treat arrhythmias according to Advanced Life Support guidelines
  - Lengthy resuscitation may be required (response may be delayed or non-existent)
  - Consider using cardiopulmonary bypass

ii) Specific Treatment: Lipid Emulsion Therapy
  - CPR must be continued throughout lipid therapy administration
  - Take blood samples in a plain and heparinized tube before and after lipid administration, and at hourly intervals, to measure LA and triglyceride levels (no interruption to CPR)
  - IV bolus injection of Intralipid® 20% 1.5ml/kg over 1 minute
  - Start an IV infusion of Intralipid® 20% at 15ml/kg/hour

- If an adequate circulation has not been restored or circulation status deteriorates after 5 minutes:
  - repeat the bolus injection twice at 5 minute intervals to maximum of three boluses
  - increase the infusion rate to 30ml/kg/hour over 10 minutes if an adequate circulation has not been restored
- Continue infusion until a stable and adequate circulation has been restored, or a maximum cumulative dose of 12ml/kg has been given

iii) Follow-up
  - Transfer to appropriate HDU or ICU care
  - Rule out pancreatitis with regular medical review and serum amylase/lipase levels for 2 days
  - Report the case to the National Patient Safety Agency, the international lipid database (http://www.lipidregistry.org), and the LipidRescue™ site (http://www.lipidrescue.org)

Notes

Reference

AAGBI. *Management of Severe Local Anaesthetic Toxicity*, AAGBI Safety Guideline. London: AAGBI, 2010

Q22 Malignant Hyperthermia

You are anaesthetising a 25-year-old woman for an emergency appendicectomy. Shortly after the operation commences, you notice the $EtCO_2$ is 7.5kPa.

a) List the causes of hypercapnia under general anaesthesia (3 marks)

b) What other factors would lead you to suspect a diagnosis of malignant hyperthermia? (3 marks)

c) Outline your immediate management of suspected malignant hyperthermia (11 marks)

d) What further clinical and non-clinical late management is required? (3 marks)

Aims

This comes under the topics of recent clinical guidelines and is easy 'examination fodder'. As with all core knowledge questions, no slip-ups would be expected. Your answer must convey your ability to correctly identify, diagnose, and manage this potentially fatal condition.

a) Causes of Hypercapnia

- Alveolar hypoventilation: obstruction, opioids, ↑ dead space (e.g. apparatus or tubing)
- Rebreathing: failure of absorption (soda lime exhaustion), inappropriate fresh gas flow
- Sepsis, ARDS
- Asthma, bronchospasm
- Hypermetabolic states: malignant hyperthermia, pyrexia, hyperthyroidism
- Inappropriate minute volume ventilation settings

b) Diagnosis of Malignant Hyperthermia

- Unexplained ↑ in $EtCO_2$, combined with:
- Unexplained ↑ in heart rate, combined with:
- Unexplained ↑ in O_2 consumption
- Presence of generalized muscle rigidity or masseter spasm

c) Immediate Management

- Call for help: assess airway, breathing whilst administering 100% O_2, circulation
- Limit the hypermetabolic process by turning off inhaled volatile agents and replacing the breathing circuit and anaesthetic machine
- Maintain anaesthesia with IV agents (e.g. propofol) and hyperventilate the patient
- Give IV dantrolene 2–3mg/kg initially, then 1mg/kg as required
- Initiate active cooling processes:
    - cold fluids and ice packs in axillae and groin
    - change active warming devices to cooling
    - cold bladder, nasogastric, and peritoneal irrigation
    - consider extracorporeal heat exchange
- Monitoring: standard AAGBI levels, invasive arterial and CVP line insertion, insert urinary catheter and measure urinary pH, measure core and peripheral temperatures
- Blood tests: arterial blood gas, FBC, U&E (to include creatine kinase), clotting
- Specific treatments:
    - IV calcium chloride or gluconate, insulin/dextrose infusion, and sodium bicarbonate if hyperkalaemic

- ◆ forced alkaline diuresis if signs of rhabdomyolysis or myoglobinuria
- ◆ blood products (e.g. packed red cells, fresh frozen plasma, platelets), cryoprecipitate if evidence of DIC
- ◆ Magnesium, amiodarone, procainamide to treat cardiac arrhythmias (Ca^{2+} blockers are contraindicated because of dantrolene interaction)

d) Further Management

- Ongoing treatment in ICU (further dantrolene therapy may be required)
- Continue to monitor for signs of renal failure, rhabdomyolysis, or compartment syndrome
- Consider differential diagnoses (e.g. recreational drugs, sepsis, endocrine tumours)
- Counselling for family
- Referral to local malignant hyperthermia unit (in Leeds for the UK)

Notes

Reference

AAGBI. *Guidelines for the Management of a Malignant Hyperthermia Crisis.* London: AAGBI, 2007

Q23 Morbid Obesity

Your next patient in pre-assessment clinic is a 42-year-old man scheduled for a right total knee replacement. His BMI is 48kg/m².

a) What are the important clinical issues to be considered for this patient at pre-assessment? (10 marks)

b) Outline the intraoperative problems presented by morbidly obese patients and how they may be managed to achieve optimal care (10 marks)

Aims

Morbid obesity is an epidemic of 'growing proportions'! It is best to divide answers into a systems-based approach followed by some technical and equipment-based issues.

a) Preoperative Assessment

- Accurate BMI calculation by measurement, and lifestyle advice on diet, exercise, and smoking
- Appropriate history, examination, and investigations to identify and optimize comorbidities
- Awareness of higher risk of comorbidities
- i) Cardiovascular System
  - Hypertension, hypercholesterolaemia, ischaemic heart disease, cardiomyopathy, heart failure
  - Thromboembolism: requires perioperative pharmacological and mechanical prophylaxis
  - ECG: ↑ risk of arrhythmias (hypertrophy, hypokalaemia 2° to diuretics, IHD, OSA, fatty infiltrates of the conducting system)
  - Consider CXR, ABG, echocardiography, CPET, pharmacological stress testing
- ii) Respiratory and Airway
  - ↑ risk of obstructive sleep apnoea, cor pulmonale (and Pickwickian syndrome), dyspnoea on exertion, and obesity hypoventilation syndrome. Consider preoperative CPAP
  - Thorough airway assessment and ability to lie supine
- iii) Gastrointestinal and Endocrine
  - ↑ risk of GORD and reflux: requires preoperative antacid treatment
  - ↑ risk of diabetes and associated complications (e.g. renal, autonomic, and cardiac): HBA1$_c$ for level of glycaemic control

b) Intraoperative Management (experienced senior anaesthetist involved)

- i) Airway
  - Appropriate airway equipment with a back-up plan. Intubation may be difficult due to deposition of fat and positioning. Allowance for potential aspiration risk: consider RSI
  - Positioning: ↓ FRC and ↑ closing volume indicates a shorter time to apnoeic desaturation during induction and airway instrumentation
  - Preoxygenation in the semi-recumbent or sitting position. 'Ramping' can improve position for successful intubation
  - Safety first: consider awake fibreoptic intubation

ii) Respiratory
   • Prone to desaturation due to shunting, hypoventilation, ↓ FRC (abdominal splinting of diaphragm), ↓ chest-wall and diaphragmatic tone, ↓ central control of hypoxia and hypercarbia
   • Difficulty in ventilation because of high peak airway pressures
   • Use of short-acting drugs is recommended (e.g. remifentanil, desflurane): ↓ risk of postoperative hypoventilation and hypoxaemia

iii) Other
   • Induction on the operating table to reduce manual handling. Consider hover mattress transfer to protect staff during manual handling
   • Choose an appropriately sized BP cuff. May require invasive monitoring (e.g. arterial line and CVP access) as cannulation can be difficult
   • Alter drug doses accordingly: ideal body weight for fat-soluble drugs (e.g. barbiturates/benzodiazepines), lean body mass for water-soluble drugs (e.g. NDMBs). Reduced LA doses for central neuraxial blocks (engorged epidural vessels/increased epidural fat content)
   • Maintain glycaemic control if diabetic: may require an insulin infusion
   • Regional anaesthetic techniques may be technically difficult or impossible, even with the additional use of ultrasound, because of excessive subcutaneous tissue

Notes

References

Lotia S, Bellamy MC. Anaesthesia and morbid obesity. *Continuing Education in Anaesthesia, Critical Care & Pain*, **8**: 151–6, 2008

AAGBI. *Peri-Operative Management of the Morbidly Obese Patient*. London: AAGBI, 2007

Q24 **Myasthenia Gravis**

A 37-year-old woman is scheduled for repair of ruptured cruciate ligaments. She is known to suffer from myasthenia gravis and has refused regional anaesthesia.

a) Define myasthenia gravis (5 marks)

b) List the signs and symptoms associated with this condition (5 marks)

c) How does the disease affect your anaesthetic management of this case? (10 marks)

Aims

Being able to incorporate core knowledge of medical conditions whilst including an understanding of the wider-ranging issues associated with safely anaesthetising these patients is a skill expected of senior anaesthetists. This question examines not only your background knowledge but also expects a considered plan and safe approach towards providing effective anaesthesia.

a) Myasthenia Gravis

- Autoimmune disease affecting mostly younger women and older men
- IgG antibodies attack acetylcholine receptors (AChR) at the post-synaptic membrane of the neuromuscular junction
- Prevents binding of ACh to its receptor, $\uparrow$ rate of AChR degradation, and stimulates complement-related damage to the post-synaptic membrane
- The 'margin of safety' is lost in neuromuscular transmission
- Associated with thymus hyperplasia in the majority of patients

b) Signs and Symptoms

- Demonstrable weakness of skeletal muscles:
  - worse post-exercise and in evening, and improved with rest
  - proximal > distal muscles
- Partial and unilateral ptosis, diplopia, blurred vision (solitary signs in 15%: ocular myasthenia gravis)
- Bulbar involvement
- Respiratory muscle involvement (20–30%), especially intercostals and diaphragm
- Sparing of sensory and reflex abnormalities
- Effects of long-term steroids (e.g. Cushingoid appearance)

c) Anaesthetic Management

i) Preoperative
- Assess bulbar and respiratory function: serial FVC measurements:
  - poor function (< 2.9L) is highly indicative of the need for postoperative ventilation
- Preoperative physiotherapy
- Optimization of anticholinesterase and immunosuppression therapy: consider plasma exchange or IV IgG if poorly controlled
- Omit anticholinesterase therapy on morning of surgery and ensure 'steroid cover' at induction if appropriate
- Premedication only in patients with good respiratory reserve

- Be aware of association with other autoimmune disease (e.g. thyroid, DM, rheumatoid arthritis)

ii) Intraoperative
- Intubation advisable as risk of aspiration is higher (bulbar involvement)
- Avoid suxamethonium: relative resistance ($\downarrow$ AChR), prolongation of action, and propensity for phase II block
- NDMBs: quicker onset and prolonged action:
  - consider intubation without NDMB (e.g. using remifentanil or volatiles)
  - reduced-dose atracurium is probably safest due to metabolism profile and avoidance of the use of neuromuscular reversal agents
- Intubation is also facilitated by exacerbated neuromuscular-blocking properties of volatile agents in myasthenia gravis

iii) Postoperative
- Extubate if uncomplicated disease state
- Have a low threshold for HDU or ICU postoperatively
- If $\downarrow$ preoperative FVC, bulbar involvement, or coexisting respiratory disease:
  - elective postoperative IPPV on ICU
  - restart anticholinesterase therapy and titrate to effect (often $\downarrow$ requirements in first 48 hours postoperatively)

Notes

Reference

Hirsch NP. Neuromuscular junction in health and disease. *British Journal of Anaesthesia* **99**: 132–8, 2007

Q25 Myotonic Dystrophy

A 32-year-old man with myotonic dystrophy is listed for a laparoscopic cholecystectomy.

a) **Outline important factors in the preoperative assessment of this patient (10 marks)**

b) **Describe your anaesthetic technique for this procedure with respect to the patient's disease (10 marks)**

Aims

Candidates must read the question in part b) carefully. It would be very easy to give a standard: 'I would give a smooth induction…' response. Relevance to the disease is important, i.e. what will prevent myotonia from occurring?

a) Preoperative Assessment

- Standard preoperative anaesthetic assessment with special attention to the following:

i) History
  - Symptoms of cardiorespiratory dysfunction (e.g. chest pain, SOB, palpitations, peripheral oedema)
  - Ask about exercise tolerance
  - Difficulties in swallowing, clearing secretions (may indicate the presence of a bulbar palsy)
  - Other comorbidities (e.g. DM, thyroid or adrenal dysfunction)

ii) Examination
  - Signs of cardiac failure
  - Mid-systolic 'click' murmur indicates mitral valve prolapse (present in 20% of patients)

iii) Investigations
  - CVS: ECG ± echocardiography (if evidence of cardiac dysfunction)
  - Respiratory: CXR, ABG ± PFTs (if evidence of respiratory dysfunction)
  - U&E and glucose
  - Premedication: antacid (e.g. ranitidine) and prokinetic (e.g. metaclopramide) as ↑ risk of aspiration (due to bulbar palsy and delayed gastric emptying)

b) Anaesthetic Techniques

- Intubation is warranted to minimize risk of aspiration of gastric contents
- Intubation without muscle relaxation is desirable (e.g. with remifentanil infusion)
- Non-depolarizing muscle relaxants have unpredictable effects; use short-acting drugs with spontaneous reversal (e.g. atracurium)
- Suxamethonium, neostigmine, and use of the peripheral nerve stimulator may precipitate myotonic contractions and should be avoided
- Consider invasive haemodynamic monitoring if cardiac dysfunction is evident
- Induction agents and high-concentration volatiles may cause significant cardiovascular instability
- Maintain adequate core body temperature with active body warming and warmed fluids to avoid shivering-induced myotonia
- Treatment of myotonia includes direct injection of LA into the muscle, phenytoin, and quinine

- Consider RA techniques to reduce postoperative opioid requirements ($\uparrow$ risk of respiratory depression)
- Postoperative management in HDU or ICU if significant cardiorespiratory history

Notes

....

....

....

....

....

....

....

....

....

....

....

Reference

Teasdale A. Dystrophia myotonica. In: Allman KG, Wilson I, eds. *Oxford Handbook of Anaesthesia* (2nd edn). Oxford University Press, 2006; 256–7

Q26 Obstructive Sleep Apnoea

The next patient in your preoperative assessment clinic is a 42-year-old man who is listed for a large epigastric hernia repair under GA. His recorded BMI is 44kg/m². His wife complains that he snores every night, occasionally 'holding his breath'.

a) What is the underlying disorder? (1 mark)

b) List predisposing factors which contribute to this disorder (6 marks)

c) Outline preoperative investigations to assess the severity of this disorder; include details of the abnormalities you would expect to see (6 marks)

d) How will the presence of this disorder affect your perioperative anaesthetic management of this patient? (7 marks)

Aims

As obesity becomes more prevalent in the UK, anaesthetists will encounter obstructive sleep apnoea more frequently. Careful directed questioning at preoperative assessment will reveal the extent of the disorder.

a) Disorder

- Obstructive sleep apnoea (OSA): described as syndrome if daytime symptoms present (e.g. somnolence)

b) Predisposing Factors

- Obesity, male gender, ↑ age, family history
- Alcohol, smoking
- Anatomical: nasal, pharyngeal (especially adeno-tonsillar hypertrophy), or laryngeal obstruction
- Craniofacial abnormalities (e.g. Pierre–Robin sequence, acromegaly, trisomy 21, mucopolysaccharide disorders)
- Other: CVA, IHD, hypertension, CRF, cerebral palsy, Cushing's syndrome, hypothyroidism

c) Preoperative Investigations

- FBC: polycythaemia
- ABG: chronic hypoxaemia, hypercapnia (including compensated metabolic state)
- ECG: right ventricular strain (right axis deviation, large P waves in II and V_1, large R wave in V_1, deep S wave in V_6), arrhythmias (e.g. AF)
- CXR: cardiomegaly, right ventricular hypertrophy, right atrial dilatation
- Echocardiogram: ↓ LV ejection fraction, right ventricular hypertrophy/dilatation, tricuspid regurgitation, ↑ pulmonary airway pressures
- Sleep studies: apnoeic periods with hypoxaemia and hypercapnia to classify type and severity of sleep disorder using EEG, EMG, respiratory measurements, and pulse oximetry

d) Perioperative Management

- Refer to sleep clinic for OSA severity assessment: may benefit from nocturnal CPAP
- If evidence of underlying CVS disease, refer to cardiology or general medicine for optimization of medical treatment

- Avoid sedative premedication
- ↑ risk of regurgitation and aspiration: preoperative antacid prophylaxis and tracheal intubation are advisable; consider RSI
- Tracheal intubation may be challenging; prepare for difficult airway management, including consideration of AFOI
- Avoid long-acting opioids: use simple analgesia (e.g. paracetamol, NSAIDs)
- Use regional anaesthesia as an adjunct; for example, rectus sheath block in this case or local infiltration where possible to avoid opioid use
- Consider postoperative HDU or ICU monitoring; may require NIV

Notes

References

Roberts F. Obstructive sleep apnoea. In: Allman KG, Wilson I, eds, *Oxford Handbook of Anaesthesia* (2nd edn). Oxford University Press, 2006; 610–11

Williams JM, Hanning CD. Obstructive sleep apnoea. *Continuing Education in Anaesthesia, Critical Care & Pain*, **3**: 75–8, 2003

Q27 Perioperative Death

During an emergency laparotomy, the patient dies from a cardiac arrest despite maximal supportive treatment

a) **Describe your initial management of the situation (13 marks)**

b) **What is the role of the anaesthetic department and the trust in subsequent management of this case? (7 marks)**

Aims

This tragic event will affect most anaesthetists in their career at some point. Whilst departmental guidelines may vary from hospital to hospital, three main points should be covered: record-keeping, communication with relatives, and organizational issues (i.e. counselling, support of clinical duties).

a) Initial Management

- Identify and contact the next of kin and request that they come to the hospital urgently
- Arrangements should be made with the nurse in charge of the patient's ward to hold a discussion in a suitable room with privacy and dignity
- Involve bereavement counsellors or nurse consultants with bereavement experience
- Contact the anaesthetic consultant on call and inform him/her of the death
- Ensure that the anaesthetic and surgical team have an opportunity to debrief and reflect
- If possible, find a colleague to take over clinical responsibilities:
  - allows time to reflect on recent events
  - focus time on coordinating the next steps required for the patient
  - removes you from working where attention may not be focused
- Whilst no formal guideline exists, most trusts have a protocol to guide duties
- Discussion with relatives is best delivered by a multidisciplinary team involving the most senior member of each team
- Begin by describing the events leading to the fact that death has occurred in a simple uncomplicated manner. Avoid the use of jargon or overcomplication
- Allow time for reflection and questioning
- Explain the process of internal investigation and requirement for referral to the coroner
- Apologizing does not imply guilt
- Do not offer opinions or hypotheses based on anything other than facts
- Consider further appointments with the next of kin; this offers the opportunity to formulate questions and clarify issues
- Detailed notes of clinical management should be made as soon as possible after the event
- A retrospective continuum detailing times, referrals, and therapies as well as copies of anaesthetic charts is invaluable
- If possible, obtain printout data from the anaesthetic machine
- All entries must be signed, legible, timed, and dated, in black ink
- Document any discussions held with the patient regarding risk and mortality
- Death during an operation mandates referral to the coroner for review
- All invasive lines, tubes, and equipment connected to the patient must be left in place
- The patient's specialty team should be informed as soon as possible of the events that have occurred
- A trust incident form must be completed

- Contact your defence union and inform them of the events that have occurred
- Make a copy of all your notes for your own records

b) Role of Anaesthetic Department and Trust

i) Role of the Anaesthetic Department
- Support for the colleague
  - Clinical: by covering shifts to allow the affected doctor time to reflect
  - Psychological: offering advice and counselling
- A senior member of the department should be allocated to act as liaison or mentor with the affected doctor
- Review of the case by the clinical director should assess the immediate risk of similar events and initiate attempts to reduce the risk
- Departmental review of the case and possible learning points should be coordinated by an individual not involved in the provision of care

ii) Role of the Trust
- Most trusts have legal and press liaison officers who should be initiated in this scenario
- Attempts to review the events and ensure that no system or operational errors contributed to the patient's death
- Most trusts have legal and press liaison officers which should be involved early if necessary

Notes

....

....

....

....

....

....

....

....

....

....

....

....

Reference

http://www.aagbi.org/publications/guidelines/docs/catastrophes05.pdf (accessed 12 November 2009)

Q28 **Phaeochromocytoma**

A 42-year-old woman is listed for a laparoscopic left adrenalectomy to remove a phaeochromocytoma.

a) **Outline the pharmacological preoperative management of this patient, giving reasons for your choice of drugs (10 marks)**

b) **What anaesthetic techniques exist to reduce cardiovascular instability during this procedure? (10 marks)**

Aims

This is a big question and tests the candidate's knowledge of cardiovascular pharmacology. Beware of misreading part b) and concentrate on specific techniques for producing cardiovascular stability.

a) Pharmacological Management

i) α-Blockers
- Used for perioperative reduction of:
  - BP
  - incidence of hypertensive crises during induction and tumour manipulation
  - myocardial dysfunction
- ↑ intravascular volume
- Stimulate resensitization of adrenergic receptors
- Perioperative aims:
  - BP <160/90 mmHg
  - orthostatic hypotension ≥80/45 mmHg
  - ischaemic-free ECG (maximum of one premature ventricular complex per 5 minutes)
  - Nasal congestion
- Non-selective: phenoxybenzamine 10mg bd (maximum 250mg/day) started 2–4 weeks prior to surgery
  - Disadvantages: α_2-blockade: tachycardia and postoperative refractory hypotension
- Selective: α_1-blockers (e.g. doxazocin, prazocin) avoid tachycardia but are less effective at preventing hypertensive crises

ii) β-Blockers
- Used to counteract tachycardia (due to α-blockers or catecholamine excess)
- Prescribed after α-blockade: avoids unopposed β_2-blockade (and resulting vasoconstriction) and ↑ risk of cardiac failure in patients with myocardial dysfunction due to ↑ afterload in combination with poor myocardial contractility
- Selective β_1-blockers (e.g. atenolol, bisoprolol) are used in COPD or PVD patients
- Non-selective (e.g. propranolol, labetalol)

b) Anaesthetic Techniques

- Aims: maintain cardiovascular stability and minimize catecholamine surges during crucial points of operation (e.g. induction and intubation, incision, tumour manipulation, post-tumour ligation and removal)
- Consider premedication to reduce anxiety and stress (e.g. temazepam, midazolam)
- Use drugs to obtund laryngoscopy pressor response (e.g. remifentanil, alfentanil, fentanyl) and ensure adequate depth of anaesthesia
- Care with histamine-releasing drugs (e.g. atracurium, morphine)

- Invasive arterial and CVP monitoring: allows accurate and quick measurement of cardiovascular status (consider TOE or PAC if severe myocardial dysfunction)
- Thoracic epidural for perioperative analgesia and sympathetic blockade
- Anaesthetic technique: avoid stimulating catecholamine release due to hypoxia, hypercarbia, pain, inadequate muscle relaxation, hypo- or hyperthermia
- Intraoperative anti-hypertensives for controlling catecholamine surges:
  - nitrates (e.g. GTN and SNP)
  - phentolamine (vasodilator and α-blocker)
  - magnesium sulphate
  - Ca^{2+}-channel blockers (e.g. nicardipine)
  - β-blockers (e.g. esmolol and labetalol (synergistic with phentolamine))
- Beware of multifactorial refractory hypotension post-tumour ligation and removal: requires fluid-loading prior to ligation ± use of vasopressors or inotropes (e.g. phenylephrine, noradrenaline, adrenaline, vasopressin)
- Post-operative: if severe comorbidities or perioperative instability, transfer to HDU or ICU to optimize cardiovascular status, fluid balance, tissue oxygenation, glycaemic control (hypoglycaemia is common problem) and analgesia

Notes

Reference

Sasidharan P, Johnston I. *Phaeochromocytoma: Perioperative Management.* Anaesthesia Tutorial Of The Week 151. Available online at: http://totw.anaesthesiologists.org (accessed 14 September 2009)

Q29 Postoperative Neuropathy

Two hours post elective laparoscopic hysterectomy, a 55-year-old woman is complaining of worsening 'pain and tingling' in her left arm.

a) List the differential diagnosis for these symptoms (6 marks)

b) Briefly explain your initial management (6 marks)

c) Describe your management of a case of suspected postoperative compression neuropathy (8 marks)

Aims

SAQs with differential diagnoses should be split into systems to allow for thoroughness. Don't forget some of the more 'medical' causes. Your management answer must cover the management and documentation issues likely to be encountered.

a) Differential Diagnoses

i) Cardiac
  * Presentation of angina or acute ischemia

ii) Central/Peripheral Nervous System
  * Migraine
  * CVA or TIA
  * Seizure phenomenon or aura
  * Perioperative brachial plexus traction injury
  * Peripheral nerve trunk compression from patient positioning
  * Compression neuropathy from repeated BP cuff inflation
  * Undiagnosed carpal tunnel syndrome
  * Compartment syndrome

iii) Respiratory
  * Hyperventilation

iv) Other
  * Thromboembolic phenomenon
  * Hypoglycaemia or hypocalcaemia
  * Local anaesthetic toxicity (although usually more central)

b) Initial Management

* Identify underlying cause
* Baseline observations reviewed and repeated
* 12-lead ECG to exclude cardiac causes
* Check blood sugar
* Systemic examination to exclude potential differentials and detect any associated symptoms or signs, including checking neurovascular status of left arm
* If metabolic or respiratory differentials, consider U&E or ABG
* If neurological cause is suspected, discussion with medical on-call team regarding management of TIA or suspected acute CVA
* Discussion with patient and explanation of likely aetiology with reassurance
* Oxygen, analgesia, anxiolytics, and IV fluids where appropriate
* Measure compartment pressure of arm if evidence of compromise
* Remain in recovery for extended period until diagnosis clearer

c) Management of Compression Neuropathy

- If expanding haematoma or vascular cause suspected: urgent imaging and surgical referral
- Evacuation of haematoma within 24 hours of onset of symptoms is associated with better recovery
- If the surgical site is involved, liaison with the surgical team is indicated urgently
- Exclusion of compartment syndrome (i.e. pain on passive movement of the limb) is an urgent priority: decompressive fasciotomy may be required
- Postoperative neuropathy is seen in 0.4% of general and 0.1% of regional cases and may present up to 14 days after surgery. Whilst positioning is usually cited, an identifiable cause is only found in <10% of cases
- Following acute and reversible causes, explanation of likely progression of injury and subsequent management is the first initial step to reassure the patient
- Development of acute pain is not uncommon and may best be managed by referral to the acute pain team
- Detailed notes of the examination, findings, and discussion with patient and other specialities
- Inform the on-call anaesthetic consultant and medical defence organisation
- Referral to a neurologist to establish diagnosis and follow up the patient, and discussion with the patient's GP informing him/her of events and future management
- Suggest an appointment with the patient in the future to allow further questions and to review progress

Notes

References

Aitkenhead AR. Complications during anaesthesia. In: Aitkenhead AR, Rowbotham AR, Smith AR, eds. *Textbook of Anaesthesia*. Edinburgh: Churchill Livingstone, 2001; 522–3

Knight DJW, Mahajan RP. Patient positioning in anaesthesia. *Continuing Education in Anaesthesia, Critical Care & Pain*, **5**: 160–3, 2004

Werrett G. Nerve injury. In: Allman KG, Wilson I., eds. *Oxford Handbook of Anaesthesia* (2nd edn). Oxford University Press, 2006; 30–3

Q30 Preoperative Assessment

a) **Outline the aims of preoperative assessment (10 marks)**

b) **Discuss the role of the anaesthetist in preoperative assessment (5 marks)**

b) **What are the benefits of a successful preoperative assessment service? (5 marks)**

Aims

This question is broad and is difficult to prepare for unless you have committed the guidelines regarding these areas to memory. Whilst reading as many of these documents before the examination is a good idea, having a system to tackle questions along these lines ensures that you usually answer much more effectively even if you forget some of the finer points.

a) Aims of Preoperative Assessment

i) For Nurses
   - To perform relevant standard investigations (e.g. blood tests, ECG, CXR)
   - Nurse assessment and information (e.g. falls assessment, go through standard questionnaire, mandatory trust requirements)
   - Information about time off, sick notes, wounds, and stitches

ii) For Doctors
   - To perform a focused medical history and examination: allows identification of pre-existing or new comorbidities
   - To identify potential anaesthetic difficulties
   - To refer for advanced investigations where appropriate (e.g. echocardiography, lung function tests, exercise stress tests, CPET)
   - To make referrals to relevant specialties (e.g. cardiologist, respiratory physicians) for preoperative optimization of comorbidities
   - To make an overall assessment of the risks faced (specifically anaesthetic and surgical) and present them to the patient, allowing the patient to make an informed decision on whether to proceed with surgery
   - To highlight any potential issues with consent (e.g. lack of capacity, learning difficulties)
   - To facilitate perioperative planning (e.g. admission the night before surgery for insulin sliding scale in diabetic patient, planning of appropriate perioperative thromboprophylaxis management in high-risk patients, postoperative HDU/ICU care)
   - To provide an opportunity to discuss anaesthetic techniques, fasting, risks, side effects: helps to reduce fear or anxiety
   - To provide lifestyle advice (e.g. losing weight, diet, smoking or alcohol reduction or cessation)
   - Overall the aim is to improve perioperative outcome and reduce the risk of adverse events. The strongest anecdotal evidence that this is the case is a reduction in 'no-shows' and cancellations, saving of money, and patients feeling that they receive a better service

b) Role of the Anaesthetist
   - Uniquely placed to provide a structure to the preoperative assessment process
   - Knowledge of anaesthetising patients with comorbidities, and what can be achieved by preoperative optimization

- Physiological and pharmacological knowledge used to assess and provide sensible and accurate advice for patients (e.g. premedication, anaesthetic techniques including regional anaesthesia and postoperative analgesia methods)
- To provide continuity on the morning of surgery, with further pre-assessment (may be different anaesthetist) of patient, discussion of precise techniques, regimens of anaesthesia and analgesia, and checking the results of any preoperative investigations or tests

c) Benefits

- Reduced rates of patient cancellation and 'no-show on the day' due to anxiety
- Reduced risk of surgery cancellation due to suboptimal control of comorbidities, lack of HDU or ICU beds, tests 'not being done'
- Increased theatre efficiency time: anaesthetic preoperative assessment is a much smoother process, so the list may start on time. Less delay in waiting for results before sending for the patient
- Financial savings and reduced cost due to the above factors
- Patient outcomes: recommended lifestyle changes (e.g. weight loss, smoking cessation, increased exercise) will not only improve perioperative outcome, but will also benefit the patient in the long term

Notes

Reference

AAGBI. *Pre-operative Assessment and Patient Preparation. The Role of the Anaesthetist 2.* AAGBI Safety Guideline. London: AAGBI, 2010

Q31 **Robotic Surgery**

A 69-year-old man is listed for a robotic-assisted laparoscopic prostatectomy.

a) **Discuss the anaesthetic-related problems that may be encountered during robot-assisted laparoscopy and how they are addressed (20 marks)**

Aims

Candidates must recognize the pitfalls of robotic surgery for the anaesthetist, namely remote access to the patient, challenging table position, and generic problems related to potentially lengthy laparoscopic surgery.

a) Problems

i) Patient Position
  - Steep Trendelenberg position and lithotomy
  - ↓ FRC, compliance, and atelectasis due to abdominal pressure on diaphragm (worse in obesity): pressure control ventilation minimizes risk of barotrauma
  - Poorly tolerated in patients with ↑ PA pressures (e.g. mitral stenosis): stimulation of pulmonary oedema due to altered position of lung relevant to left atrium
  - Careful eye protection required to protect from gastric secretions and robotic instruments
  - ↑ risk of cerebral oedema: requires tight ventilatory $EtCO_2$ control and cautious intraoperative fluid administration (will also obstruct surgical field of vision because of excessive urine output)
  - Rapid assessment and wake-up is necessary at the end: short-acting agents (e.g. desflurane, remifentanil) are desirable
  - Facial oedema: if significant may indicate upper airway oedema and potential difficulties post-extubation (e.g. obstruction or inability to re-intubate). Perform tracheal cuff-leak test; patient should remain intubated until oedema has subsided
  - Upward movement of trachea: endobroncheal intubation (exacerbated by insufflation of pneumoperitoneum); ensure regular checks of tracheal tube position
  - ↑ risk of neuropraxia: in lower limbs due to lithotomy and in upper limbs due to incorrect use of shoulder braces. Careful positioning and padding of pressure areas required pre-surgery

ii) CO_2 Pneumoperitoneum
  Cardiovascular System
  - ↑ CVP, PAP, SVR, MAP, HR (may ↓ with vagal stretch) and ↓ cardiac output
  - Altered parameters normally tolerated in healthy patients but may precipitate myocardial ischaemia or pulmonary oedema in those with cardiac disease
  - Invasive monitoring is recommended, including CVP in patients with evidence of cardiovascular dysfunction
  - ↑ afterload is treated with inhalational agents, nitrates, or α_2-agonist (e.g. clonidine)
  Respiratory System
  - ↑V/Q mismatch, airway pressures and ↓compliance, FRC, VC
  - Hypercarbia: risk of CVS instability (e.g. hypertension, arrhythmias) and cerebral oedema (due to vasodilatation) minimized by altering ventilator parameters to maintain normocapnia

Other
- Regurgitation and aspiration of gastric contents: tracheal intubation and nasogastric tube should be mandatory for this procedure, and preoperative antacid and prokinetic therapy should be prescribed
- Risk of venous air embolism (laparoscopic procedure and operation site above cardiac level): be aware of sudden CVS collapse and consider arterial embolism (20% of patients have a patent foramen ovale). Requires deflation of pneumoperitoneum and supportive treatment if suspected

iii) The Robot
- Space and anaesthetic access intraoperatively will be limited due to the size of the machinery and the nature of robotic surgery, i.e. multiple ports in abdomen and pelvis
- Ensure that the tracheal tube, adequate venous and arterial access, line extensions, body warmers, core temperature monitoring, and pressure area and venothromboembolism protection devices are well secured prior to starting surgery
- The patient must remain motionless intraoperatively; movement or coughing could be disastrous because of the fixed ports in the abdomen. Continuous monitoring and an infusion of non-depolarizing muscle relaxant ± remifentanil are the most common methods used

Notes

References

Baltayian S. A brief review: anesthesia for robotic prostatectomy. *Journal of Robotic Surgery*, **2**: 59–66, 2008

Irvine M, Patil V. Anaesthesia for robot-assisted laparoscopic surgery. *Continuing Education in Anaesthesia, Critical Care & Pain*, **9**, 125–9

Q32 **Rocuronium and Sugammadex**

a) **Compare and contrast vecuronium and rocuronium related to their clinical applications (10 marks)**

b) **Describe classes of drugs used to reverse the effect of rocuronium, including an explanation of their mechanism of action (10 marks)**

Aims

Sugammadex is a novel drug and thus is a trendy topic for the Final FRCA examination, having appeared once already in the written SAQ section. As more data and evidence for its use surface, it will continue to be an important topic to be aware of.

a) Vecuronium and Rocuronium

	Vecuronium	Rocuronium
Class	Monoquaternary aminosteroid	Monoquaternary aminosteroid
Presentation	Lipophilized white powder	Clear colourless solution
Dose, speed of onset	0.1mg/kg, 2min	0.6mg/kg, 2–3min
		1.2mg/kg, <1min
Duration of action	20–35min	20–35min
Relative potency	1	0.15
Volume of distribution	0.2L/kg	0.2L/kg
Protein binding	60–90%	30%
Metabolism	Hepatic–active metabolites	Nil
Excretion	25% unmetabolized in urine	40% unmetabolized in bile
	20% unmetabolized in bile	15% unmetabolized in urine
Clearance	3–6.4mL/kg/min	3.9mL/kg/min
Effect of increasing dose	↑ duration of relaxation	↑ speed of onset

- Rocuronium is the monoquaternary derivative of vecuronium
- Speed of onset is inversely proportional to potency; therefore a low-potency drug will have a faster speed of onset. This is due to the relative increase in the number of drug molecules required to produce the same clinical effect
- Rocuronium's lower potency and lower plasma protein binding allows more rapid access to the neuromuscular junction (NMJ) and, by increasing the dose, explains why it is possible to achieve rapid-onset neuromuscular blockade more effectively than with vecuronium
- Duration of action is related to the ligand receptor binding affinity. An avidly bound ligand will produce clinical effects for longer than one that easily dissociates

b) Reversal of Rocuronium

- Either by competitive agonism of normal physiological mechanisms or chelation methods
- Termination of effect following a bolus of NDMB is due to diffusion of the drug away from the NMJ, reducing the number of pre- and post-synaptic receptors blocked

i) Competitive Reversal
  - Infusion of neostigmine prevents the breakdown of acetylcholine (ACh), ↑ the probability of Ach displacing a NDMB and triggering an excitatory post-synaptic potential

- Works by reversibly complexing with the esteratic site of acetylcholinesterase, preventing the breakdown of ACh
- Given with glycopyrrolate to attenuate muscarinic effects caused by excessive ACh accumulation (M_2, bradycardia; M_3, excessive GI secretions)
- Onset is 4–6min after administration; this is why glycopyrrolate is given, as the onset and duration of the two drugs are similar
- If atropine is used, an initial tachycardia and late bradycardia may manifest because of its faster speed of onset and shorter duration of action

ii) Chelation
- Sugammadex, trade name Bridion
- Selective relaxant binding agonist (SRBA)
- Modified γ-cyclodextrin which contains a high density of negative charge to attract the positive amino moieties within NDMB
- High-affinity bond renders rocuronium inactive; cleared renally without hepatic metabolism
- Most studies have investigated reversal of rocuronium, although reversal effects on vecuronium and pancuronium are documented; usual dose 4mg/kg
- Found to produce reversal of neuromuscular blockade rapidly at a dose of 16mg/kg (1.3–1.8min) following RSI with rocuronium 1.2mg/kg
- Cochrane Review found it to be more effective at reversal of NDMB with a lower incidence of side effects (reports of anaphylaxis and prolonged QT are documented)
- Theoretical late release of drug is possible if other positively charged drugs displace rocuronium, or in patients with reduced renal clearance
- Repeat anaesthesia within 24 hours will require non-aminosteroid muscle relaxation

Notes

References

Abrishami A., Ho J, Wong J, Chin L, Chung F. Sugammadex, a selective reversal medication for preventing postoperative residual neuromuscular blockade." *Cochrane Database System Review*, **4**: CD007362, 2009

Pühringer FK, Rex C, Sielenkämper AW, *et al*. Reversal of profound, high-dose rocuronium-induced neuromuscular blockade by sugammadex at two different time points: an international, multicenter, randomized, dose-finding, safety assessor-blinded, phase II trial. *Anesthesiology*, **109**: 188–97, 2008

http://www.bridion.com (accessed 24 January 2010)

Q33 Severe Hypertension

Whilst anaesthetising a 55-year-old man for repair of left inguinal hernia under general anaesthesia, you notice that his BP reading is 225/115mmHg

a) List the potential causes for hypertension in this case (5 marks)

b) Describe your immediate management, including any appropriate pharmacological interventions (10 marks)

c) What secondary management options or investigations would be indicated? (5 marks)

Aims

This is a potentially realistic scenario that should be swiftly recognized, diagnosed, and treated appropriately by competent candidates. Calling for help and ABC management are mandatory for success in this question.

a) Causes of Hypertension

i) Anaesthetic
  * Equipment or measurement error
  * Pain (including tourniquet cuff)
  * Hypoxia or hypercarbia
  * Inadequate depth of anaesthesia or muscle relaxation
  * Drug error (type, dose, concentration, route of delivery)

ii) Patient
  * Raised intracranial pressure
  * Thyroid storm
  * Phaeochromocytoma
  * Malignant Hypertension

iii) Surgical
  * Cross-clamping of major vessels in vascular surgery

b) Immediate Management

* Stop surgery; airway, breathing, circulation; 100% O_2, *call for help*
* Repeat NIBP, ensuring cuff size and site is appropriate and no movement artefact
* If invasive arterial BP monitoring, check transducer height, check cannula site for kinking or blockage, and flush system to remove air bubbles (not into patient!)
* If tourniquet present and inflated, ask surgeon to deflate cuff
* Check position of ETT or patency of LMA and ability to ventilate manually
* Adjust minute volume ventilation to correct hypercarbia if ↑EtCO$_2$. Obtain an arterial blood gas sample to assess PaCO$_2$ if ↑ A–a gradient suspected, i.e. pulmonary disease
* ↑ volatile agent concentration and fresh gas flow delivery; if using TIVA, check the cannula site and flush for patency of line. If necessary, ↑ infusion rates
* Administer further non-depolarizing muscle relaxant if evidence of spontaneous ventilation
* If pain suspected: administer a further bolus of opiate or ↑ remifentanil infusion
* Re-check recent drugs administered (e.g. LA with adrenaline, Moffet's solution with cocaine). Check patient's notes for past drug history (e.g. MAOI interactions with ephedrine)

- If ↑ ICP suspected: check pupil size and response to light; maintain 30° head-up tilt; aim for MAP >80mmHg, normocarbia, and PaO_2 >13kPa; avoid venous obstruction; consider IV mannitol 0.5g/kg
- Further pharmacological interventions
  - GTN: initially two sprays sublingually, then an infusion of 1mg/ml titrated to BP
  - Magnesium sulphate: 2–4g bolus over 15 minutes then 1g/hour infusion
  - Hydralazine: 5mg IV bolus, repeated every 15 minutes
  - Labetalol: 5–10mg IV bolus, titrated to effect
  - Consider phentolamine in severe cases: 1mg IV bolus, titrated to effect

c) Secondary Management Options

- Arrange HDU/ICU transfer for postoperative care if the patient remains unstable
- Rule out cardiac ischaemia: 12-lead ECG, troponin levels, and echocardiography if appropriate
- If ↑ ICP suspected, perform CT head and refer to neurosurgeons if appropriate
- If thyroid storm suspected, treat with β-blockade, steroids, and propylthiouracil (to suppress thyroid hormone release and peripheral conversion). Check postoperative thyroid function test and refer to endocrinologist for optimization of disease
- If phaeochromocytoma suspected, send 24 hour urinary catecholamines. Investigations include meta-iodobenzylguanidine (MIBG) scan, MRI, and contrast CT (only in α/β-blocked patients because of the risk of crisis provocation). Refer to physicians/surgeons specializing in phaeochromocytoma management

Notes

Reference

McIndoe A. Anaesthetic emergencies. In: Allman KG, Wilson IH, eds (2nd edn). *Oxford Handbook Of Anaesthesia*. Oxford University Press, 2006; 872–3

Q34 Surgical Safety Checklist

a) **In a hospital trust, who is responsible for implementing and maintaining a surgical safety checklist? (5 marks)**

b) **What are the important factors to be discussed:**

   i) **prior to anaesthetic induction? (5 marks)**

   ii) **prior to surgical incision? (5 marks)**

   iii) **at the end of the surgical procedure? (5 marks)**

Aims

With most hospitals adopting the use of the perioperative WHO checklist, this should be a gift question. Just think back to the previous day's surgery! Questions along this line are increasingly occurring in the examination and therefore should be integrated into your revision.

a) Responsibility

- All staff involved with the patient's care throughout the perioperative pathway
- An executive at board level and a clinical lead are appointed to implement the surgical safety checklist
- Ward staff and porters who prepare and accompany the patient to theatre
- The anaesthetist and ODP or anaesthetic nurse
- The surgeon and surgical assistants
- The appointed theatre clinical lead for the day
- Theatre scrub staff, healthcare assistants, auxiliaries, runners
- Theatre manager, clinical lead
- Recovery staff

b) Surgical Safety Checklist

   i) Prior to Anaesthetic Induction
   - Confirm that the correct patient is having the correct surgery at the correct site
   - Confirm that consent for surgery has been obtained by the surgeon, and that the correct type of consent form has been filled out and signed correctly
   - Check that the surgical site has been marked, if appropriate
   - Confirm that anaesthetic machines, equipment, and drugs have been checked and are prepared adequately according to known guidelines
   - Identify patients at risk of above-average blood loss during the procedure (i.e. >500mL or 7mL/kg in children)
   - Identify patients with a potentially difficult airway or a high risk of aspiration
   - Reconfirm any patient allergies

   ii) Prior to surgical incision
   - All theatre team members to introduce themselves by name and role
   - Reconfirm the patient's name, procedure, site, and position prior to incision
   - Highlight any procedure-specific equipment or investigations required
   - Ensure that appropriate imaging devices with trained personnel are available
   - Confirm the sterility of all surgical instruments and equipment
   - Highlight any anticipated or potential critical incidents:
     - expected blood loss and potential need for blood products

- patient-specific concerns, i.e. co-morbidities, ASA grading, monitoring equipment, levels of support required
- equipment issues
- Confirm that surgical site infection prophylaxis has occurred, if appropriate:
  - antibiotic prophylaxis within 60 minutes prior to incision
  - adequate glycaemic control
  - hair removal
  - patient warming
- Confirm that venous thromboembolism prophylaxis has occurred

iii) At the end of the surgical procedure
- Check that the procedure has been adequately and correctly recorded
- Confirm that all instrument, swab, and sharps counts are complete
- Confirm that all specimens are labelled and packaged correctly
- Identify any equipment issued that should be addressed
- Highlight major concerns for the post-operative management and recovery of the patient

Notes

....

....

....

....

....

....

....

....

....

....

....

Reference

National Patient Safety Agency (NPSA). *WHO Surgical Safety Checklist*. Available online at: http://www.nrls.npsa.nhs.uk/resources/clinical-specialty/surgery/?entryid45=59860 (accessed 25 October 2009)

Q35 Thromboelastography

a) Explain the principle behind the function of a thromboelastography (TEG) machine (4 marks)

b) Define the following parameters obtained from a TEG: R-time, K-time, α-angle, MA, and Ly30 (9 marks)

c) Draw the TEG pattern generated in the following situations and list the abnormal components associated with each diagram (7 marks)

   i)   Presence of anticoagulants

   ii) Presence of antiplatelet agents or thrombocytopenia

   iii) DIC stages 1 and 2

Aims

This simple bedside investigation can be invaluable in diagnosing and managing a bleeding patient. Candidates should be able to interpret TEGs and initiate appropriate treatment based on their findings.

a) TEG Machine

- Thromboelastography is a bedside analysis of clotting performed on whole blood which produces quick results on both the quality and speed of clot formation
- A small sample (<0.5ml) of whole blood is introduced into a rotating and oscillating cup in which a wire sits
- As the blood clot thickens, movements of the cup are transmitted via the wire and translated into a graphical output which correlates with the viscoelastic properties of the clot formed
- The advantage of TEG is that it provides information on both the strength of the clot formed and fibrinolysis, neither of which are assessed using APTT or PT

b) TEG Parameters

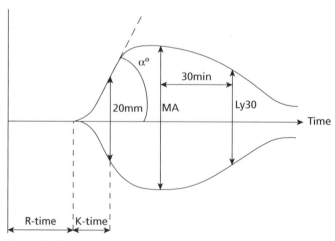

Figure 3. Thromboelastography

i) R-Time
- Time taken from start of test to initial fibrin formation (1mm). This correlates with APTT and PT.

ii) K-Time
- Time taken for graph to widen to 20mm. Represents dynamics of clot formation and depends on fibrinogen formation and platelet function

iii) α-Angle
- Angle measured between the midline of the tracing and a line drawn from 1mm point tangential to the curve. Represents acceleration of fibrin build-up and cross-linking

iv) Maximum Amplitude (MA)
- Represents ultimate strength of the clot and depends on number and function of platelets and time

v) Lysis (Ly30)
- Measures percentage of amplitude reduction 30 minutes after the MA. Indicates the stability of the clot

c) Abnormal TEG Traces

i) Anticoagulants
- ↑ R-time and K-time
- ↓ MA and α-angle

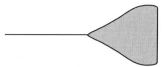

Figure 4. Anticoagulants

ii) Antiplatelet agents/thrombocytopenia
- Normal R-time
- ↑ K-time
- ↓ MA

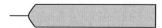

Figure 5. Antiplatelet agents

iii) DIC

Stage 1: Hypercoagulable state and 2° Fibrinolysis
- ↓ R-time and K-time
- ↑ α-angle and MA (then continuous ↓)
- Ly30 >7.5% and Ly60 >15%

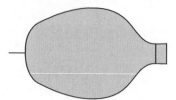

Figure 6. DIC stage 1

Stage 2: Hypocoagulable State
- As for i) but ↓MA

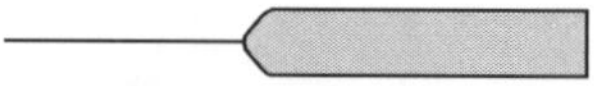

Figure 7. DIC stage 2

Notes

Q36 **Throat Packs**

a) List the reasons for inserting a throat pack during surgery (4 marks)

b) Outline procedures which exist to reduce the risk of postoperative throat pack retention (10 marks)

c) What complications may arise from the use of a throat pack? (6 marks)

Aims

The importance of reading national guidelines (e.g. NPSA, NICE) is highlighted by this relatively straightforward SAQ appearing in a recent sitting of the examination.

a) Reasons for Insertion

- To absorb any surgical debris or material from the mouth
- To prevent blood, fluids, or surgical debris from entering the lungs or oesophagus
- To reduce the leak of exhaled anaesthetic gases from around an endotracheal tube
- To stabilise supraglottic airways, especially in the edentulous patient

b) Risk Reduction

i) Visual Checks
- A portion of the throat pack is left external from the mouth where it can be seen
- An easily visible mark is made on the patient (e.g. the head, neck, or sternum) using tape or stickers
- An easily visible label is made on the endotracheal tube or supraglottic device
- A visible label is attached to the anaesthetic machine
- The throat pack is securely tied or taped to the airway device
- A verbal statement is made by the surgeon or anaesthetist to confirm removal of the throat pack

ii) Written Checks
- Protocol-driven 'double check', i.e. two staff members to confirm insertion and removal of throat pack: recorded and inserted into the patient's notes or surgical care plan
- Incorporate throat pack management into a safe surgical checklist, i.e. recording of throat pack insertion, removal with swab, sharps count

c) Complications

i) During insertion
- Injury to lips, tongue, frenulum, soft palate
- Dental damage
- Uvula laceration

ii) Postoperatively
- Airway obstruction: can lead to hypoxia, negative-pressure pulmonary oedema, and ultimately coma and death
- Dysphagia
- Sore throat postoperatively

Notes

Reference

National Patient Safety Agency. *Throat Packs.* Available online at: http://www.nrls.npsa.nhs.uk/
resources/?entryid45=59853 (accessed 4 November 2009)

Q37 Thyroidectomy

A 43-year-old woman is listed for a total thyroidectomy. She has a significant goitre secondary to Graves' disease. Relevant to *this surgery*

a) What are the important factors which must be covered in the preoperative assessment? (5 marks)

b) Outline specific intraoperative considerations in anaesthetic technique, including induction (8 marks)

c) List potential postoperative complications and briefly explain how they can be prevented or treated (7 marks)

Aims

The CEACCP articles included every other month with the *British Journal of Anaesthesia* are used as subjects for both the SAQ and SOE section of the examination time and time again. Part of your revision for this examination should be the review of at least a year's worth of CEACCP topics.

a) Preoperative Assessment

- History: airway and respiratory symptoms (e.g. positional dyspnoea (especially when lying flat), hoarse voice, stridor)
- Symptoms of hyper- or hypothyroidism: aim is for euthyroid state clinically and biochemically
- Examination: airway, goitre, trachea (deviation or retrosternal extension), SVC obstruction, stridor, thyroid signs (as above), neck movement range (requires extension for surgery)
- Investigations: FBC, U&Es, corrected Ca^{2+}, TFTs in normal range
- Imaging: traditionally CXR with thoracic inlet view. Now CT is used to determine size, spread, and encroachment of thyroid gland on airway
- Vocal cord check: via nasendoscopy (LA) either preoperatively by an ENT surgeon, or pre-induction by the anaesthetist (see later)

b) Intraoperative Considerations

i) Airway Management
- Usually standard IV induction and intubation (reinforced ETT), preferably in sitting or semi-recumbent position
- If significant stridor or obstruction, consider inhalational induction with sevoflurane
- Awake fibreoptic intubation (beware 'cork-in-bottle' obstruction in stridulous patient) in distorted laryngeal anatomy or neck pathology
- Tracheostomy (LA) only if access to trachea inferior to obstruction
- Ventilation through rigid bronchoscope if unable to pass ETT past obstruction
- Vocal cord check: LA to nasal cavity and oropharynx, and fibreoptic bronchoscopy to assess vocal cord function (medico-legal considerations)

ii) Perioperative
- Eyes taped and padded, especially if exophthalmos present
- Neck extended with table in reverse Trendelenberg position to aid surgical access and allow adequate venous drainage

- Ensure adequate relaxation: peripheral neuromuscular monitoring and a bolus of NDMB or consider remifentanil infusion (see later)
- Dexamethasone 8mg IV: ↓ risk of postoperative oedema and antiemesis

iii) Analgesia
- Bilateral superficial cervical plexus blocks post-induction
- Consider remifentanil infusion
- Paracetamol and NSAIDs; stronger opiates infrequent if successful RA

c) Postoperative Complications

- Post-extubation respiratory obstruction or stridor: ABC with 100% O_2 approach
  - If extreme, re-intubate and ventilate; may need tracheostomy if severe
  - Recurrent laryngeal nerve palsy or tracheomalacia assessed in recovery with awake patient in sitting position
- Expanding haematoma: may cause airway obstruction and/or respiratory distress. Remove skin clips and underlying sutures to evacuate clot at bedside or in theatre
- Hypocalcaemia (due to parathyroid excision): if serum Ca^{2+} >2.0mmol/L administer postoperative oral Ca^{2+} supplements; if serum Ca^{2+} <2.0mmol/L give 10mL 10% calcium gluconate IV over 10 minutes and prescribe PO alfacalcidol or dihydroxycholecalciferol 1–5g
- Pneumothorax: if retrosternal thyroid dissection and thoracotomy. CXR in recovery
- Rarely, thyroid crisis: treat with β-blockers, steroids, and thyroid-suppression therapy in high-dependency care

Notes

References

Batchelor A. Thyroidectomy. In: Allman KG, Wilson I, eds. *Oxford Handbook of Anaesthesia* (2nd edn). Oxford University Press, 2006; 554–7

Malhotra S, Sodhi V. Anaesthesia for thyroid and parathyroid surgery. *Continuing Education in Anaesthesia, Critical Care & Pain*, **7**: 55–7, 2007

Q38 Total Intravenous Anaesthesia

a) Outline i) the advantages (7 marks) and ii) the disadvantages (7 marks) of using total intravenous anaesthesia (TIVA)

b) What recommendations exist to prevent critical incidents occurring during TIVA use? (6 marks)

Aims

You should be able to explain common systems used to deliver TIVA systems, as well as the pharmacological models behind their use and the drugs used. As with any system, a unique set of complications exist and an awareness of these will help to minimize their chance of occurring.

a) TIVA

i) Advantages
   - Useful for patients at high risk of postoperative nausea and vomiting
   - Used in patients with a history or family history of malignant hyperthermia
   - Used to maintain anaesthesia where volatile anaesthetic delivery may be unreliable or difficult (e.g. bronchoscopy, laryngoscopy, shared-airway surgery)
   - Ability to instrument the airway without muscle relaxation
   - Smoother recovery profile: useful where there should be minimal or no coughing or straining on the tracheal tube at extubation (may exacerbate bleeding) (e.g. middle-ear or nasal surgery)
   - Maintenance of anaesthesia without lung ventilation (e.g. during cardiac bypass surgery)
   - Useful in neurosurgery: $\downarrow$ ICP 2° to $\downarrow$ cerebral metabolic rate of O_2 (CMRo_2)
   - Decreased atmospheric pollution compared with volatiles: no gaseous by-products
   - Potential (controversial) advantage during one-lung surgery because of preservation of HPV (compared with volatiles which uncouple HPV, worsening V/Q mismatch

ii) Disadvantages
   - More expensive than volatile anaesthesia: specific equipment and drugs, including a controlled drug (further potential for drug errors or abuse)
   - Requires specific training and understanding of pharmacokinetics and pharmacodynamics
   - Difficult to alter depth of anaesthesia quickly; relies on patient pharmacokinetics (i.e. redistribution and elimination of drug)
   - Inability to monitor effectiveness of anaesthesia accurately; effect site concentrations are calculated using complex mathematics
   - Occasionally difficulty in ventilation with remifentanil
   - Risk of awareness is higher (e.g. due to kinking or blocking of infusion tubing, loss of IV access, disconnections, failure of equipment)
   - May be cardiovascularly unstable in susceptible patients (e.g. sepsis, CVS disease, elderly)

b) Recommendations
   - Use a one-way valve on the IV fluid port when multi-lumen IV connectors are used
   - All packaging for one-way valves must be clearly labelled to ensure that the correct infusion equipment is selected for TIVA use

- Continual monitoring and vigilance regarding IV access site, infusion pumps, and infusion lines must be maintained during the case
- Trusts must ensure that all infusion pumps are maintained in working condition and service regularly
- All clinicians should be expected to ensure they have had adequate training in all aspects of TIVA. Trainees should undergo competency testing, signed by more than one consultant, prior to solo use of TIVA

Notes

Reference

Safe Anaesthesia Liaison Group. *Guaranteeing Drug Delivery in Total Intravenous Anaesthesia*. London: National Patient Safety Agency, 2009

Q39 Tourniquet

a) **Describe the systemic effects of tourniquet use (6 marks)**

b) **List the contraindications to using an arterial tourniquet in surgery (6 marks)**

c) **What local complications may occur? (8 marks)**

Aims

The consequences of ischaemic reperfusion injury should not be underestimated. The benefits of improved operative field, reduced blood loss, and consequential shorter operation times should not persuade you to use a device that may prove to be a fatal error at the end of a shorter bloodless operation.

a) Systemic Effects

i) Post-inflation
- $\uparrow$SVR $\rightarrow \uparrow$ circulating volume $\rightarrow \uparrow$ CVP and initial $\uparrow$ BP
- Slower gradual $\uparrow$ in BP over time, probably 2° to tourniquet pain
- Induced hypercoagulable state due to catecholamine-induced platelet aggregation
- Slow $\uparrow$ in core body temperature because of lack of heat transfer in limb

ii) Post-deflation
- $\downarrow$ CVP and BP 2° to blood volume and cold ischaemic metabolite distribution
- $\uparrow$ EtCO$_2$ due to $\uparrow$ mixed venous Pvco$_2$ and $\uparrow$ cardiac output (2° to $\downarrow$ BP)
- $\uparrow$ EtCO$_2$ $\rightarrow \uparrow$ cerebral blood flow and $\uparrow$ ICP (detrimental in head injury patients)
- Enhanced fibrinolysis: $\uparrow$ plasminogen activator release in a hypoxic acidotic limb
- $\downarrow$ core body temperature due to redistribution of cold acidotic blood
- Metabolic changes: $\uparrow$ plasma K$^+$, lactate, O$_2$ consumption, CO$_2$ production, $\downarrow$ pH

b) Contraindications

i) Absolute
- AV fistula
- Severe peripheral vascular disease
- Previous vascular surgery to limb
- Evidence of bone fracture or thrombosis at the proposed tourniquet site

ii) Relative
- Sickle cell disease (requires pre-optimization of analgesia, oxygenation, hydration, and temperature before use)
- History of thromboembolic disease
- Skin grafts
- Localized infection
- Lymphoedema e.g. secondary to axillary clearance after breast cancer surgery and radiotherapy

c) Local Complications

i) Damage to Skin
- Friction if tourniquet applied incorrectly
- Chemical burn: leakage of alcohol skin preparation beneath tourniquet

ii) Damage to Muscle
   - Swelling, oedema, and hyperaemia
   - Rarely, rhabdomyolysis and/or compartment syndrome
   - 2° to high cuff inflation pressures or extended ischaemic limb time

iii) Damage to Vessels
   - Patients with arterial vascular disease are more susceptible because of atheromatous plaque rupture
   - May be severe enough to require amputation

iv) Damage to Nerves
   - ↑ risk with: extended limb ischaemic time, poorly applied tourniquet, and direct neurological pressure effect
   - Motor function affected more than sensory function (large-diameter nerve fibres are more susceptible to injury)
   - Lower limb affected more than upper limb

Notes

Reference

Deloughry JL, Griffiths R. Arterial tourniquets. *Continuing Education in Anaesthesia, Critical Care & Pain*, **9**: 56–60, 2009

Q40 **Trial Design**

You are part of a group designing a new analgesic drug for routine postoperative use.

a) Describe the stages used in the development and introduction of this new drug to clinical practice (13 marks)

b) Define type 1 and 2 errors and statistical power (7 marks)

Aims

Statistics and study design are traditionally disliked by candidates. However, the type of potential question is finite and should not be ignored as statistics does occur regularly in the SAQ paper.

a) Drug Trials

i) Initial stages
   - Product design and development
   - Literature review to identify previous data that may alter the final product, i.e. similar research and other novel products. Observational studies may exist already
   - Involves market research to identify competing interests and suitability for drug development
   - May alter design of product, trial, or overall aim of the study

ii) Pilot study
   - Meet with statistician to identify numbers needed for adequate power and significance
   - Identify hypothesis and how it will be tested
   - Apply for ethical approval: register with IRAS (Integrated Research Application System)
   - IRAS requires information on
     - study: design, methodology, statistical analysis
     - logistical structures, i.e. where the trial will be conducted and who is involved
     - background data: results of the literature review
     - safety: possible risks and example of patient information leaflet used in the trial

iii) Phase 0
   - Animal studies to identify the median lethal dose (LD_{50}) and the 95% lethal dose (LD_{95})

iv) Phase 1
   - The drug is administered to small groups of *healthy* volunteers (<100)
   - Aims to identify pharmacological traits, i.e. activity, tolerance, pharmacokinetics, safety
   - Can also identify potential routes by which the drug can be administered
   - Performed in a safe clinical setting where subjects can be monitored for both side effects and desired response to the drug

v) Phase 2
   - First stage where drug is administered to patients with the disease/condition
   - Usually of magnitude of hundreds
   - Aim is to identify ED_{50} (dose that produces desired effect in half the population) and ED_{95}
   - Can now involve specialists in the chosen field to assess the clinical effects of the drug

vi) Phase 3
   - Only able to commence after satisfactory phase 2 trials completed

- Extended clinical trials involving large (usually thousands) numbers of patients in multiple-site double-blind randomized controlled trials (DBRCTs)
- Aim is to compare drug with 'gold standard' therapy currently available in an attempt to identify superiority, identify efficacy, and ensure that side effects and adverse reactions occur at an acceptable rate

vii) Phase 4
  - Post-marketing analysis
  - Often this stage is when most adverse reactions are detected because of the statistical power created by large numbers of drug administrations
  - Adverse events are recorded by prescribers via the yellow sheets in the BNF
  - No fixed duration for this stage

b) Error and Power

i) Type 1 (or α) Error
  - A 'false-positive' result
  - Incorrectly rejecting a null hypothesis when it is actually true: states that a difference is observed when there isn't one present
  - Determined by the p value
  - Smaller p values $\downarrow$ the chance of type 1 error

ii) Type 2 (or β) Error
  - A 'false-negative' result
  - Incorrectly accepting a null hypothesis when it is not true: fails to observe a difference when there is one present
  - Usually a result of small sample size

iii) Power
  - Refers to the ability of a study to reject a false null hypothesis, i.e. not make a type 2 error
  - Power = 1 − probability of type 2 (β) error = sensitivity
  - Routinely, β is accepted as 0.2, i.e. there is a 20% chance of the null hypothesis being falsely accepted
  - Therefore power is usually accepted at a level of 80%
  - Power calculations are performed in the initial stages of trial design to help identify the trial numbers required to detect a result and reduce the chance that type 2 errors will occur
  - Importance of having a highly powered study includes:
    - $\downarrow$ the chance of α and β errors
    - $\uparrow$ the chance of finding a result
    - detecting a result if it is present
    - preventing unnecessary exposure of patient groups to repeated trials

Notes

Q41 Venous Air Embolism

a) Describe the clinical features of a massive venous air embolism (VAE) (10 marks)

b) Describe your immediate management of a suspected VAE during a laparoscopic hemicolectomy (10 marks)

Aims

Thankfully, this is an uncommon anaesthetic emergency; however it frequents the FRCA examination disproportionately. Divide the features into a systems-based approach.

a) Clinical Features

i) Symptoms (awake patients only)
   - Dizziness, light-headedness, vertigo
   - Nausea
   - Agitation
   - SOB and cough (feature of pulmonary oedema with pink frothy sputum)
   - 'Gasp' reflex (bolus of air entering pulmonary circulation, causing acute hypoxaemia)
   - Substernal chest pain

ii) Signs

Cardiovascular
   - Dysrrhythmias (tachy- more than bradyarrythmias)
   - 'Mill wheel' murmur
   - Pulmonary artery hypertension
   - Myocardial ischaemia, non-specific ST-segment and T-wave changes and/or evidence of right heart strain ± jugular distension
   - Circulatory shock, cardiovascular collapse, hypotension

Respiratory
   - Tachypnoea, haemoptysis, wheeze, cyanosis
   - Abnormal capnography, $\downarrow$ EtCO$_2$
   - $\uparrow$ PaCO$_2$, $\downarrow$ PaO$_2$
   - Pulmonary oedema

Neurological
   - Owing to shock or in the presence of a patent foramen ovale, gas bubbles enter the arterial circulation and occlude arterial inflow within the cerebral circulation causing:
     - acute confusion
     - seizures
     - transient or permanent focal deficits (weakness, paraesthesias, paralysis)
     - coma

b) Initial Management
   - Recognize diagnosis, ABC, 100% O$_2$, and call for help
   - Inform surgeon of diagnosis. Attempt to $\downarrow$ volume and rate of gas entrainment by:
     - deflating pneumoperitoneum immediately
     - flooding the surgical site with saline
   - If used, switch N$_2$O to air (expansion of bubbles due to accumulation of N$_2$O)
   - Use PEEP and IV fluid administration to $\uparrow$ venous pressure and $\downarrow$ entrainment into venous circulation

- If cardiac arrest occurs, initiate CPR in a supine head-down position (cardiac massage may help break large bubbles into smaller fragments)
- Turning patient into left lateral position (Durant manoeuvre) may:
  - ◆ ↓ the amount of blood accumulating within the right ventricle
  - ◆ ↓ the volume of air ejected into the pulmonary circulation
  - ◆ ↑ the right ventricle stroke volume
  - ◆ allow air to accumulate within the apex of the right ventricle to aid aspiration
- Insert a right internal jugular line and attempt to aspirate air which may be present in the right ventricle
- Continue fluids; insert arterial line – may require inotropes
- Terminate surgery and transfer to ICU for further stabilization and investigation
- Assess severity: may require transfer to hyperbaric oxygen chamber:
  - ◆ ↓ size of bubbles already present
  - ◆ speed up bubble resolution in circulation: establishes high diffusion gradient
  - ◆ ↑ dissolved oxygen content to improve oxygen delivery to tissue
  - ◆ shown to ↓ mortality in patients with cerebral air emboli
- Experimental data from animal models have shown that the use of perfluorocarbons (FP43) aids the dissolution of gas bubbles

Notes

References

Mirski MA, Lele AV, Fitzsimmons L, Toung TJ. Diagnosis and treatment of vascular air embolism. *Anesthesiology*, **106**: 164–77, 2007

Sviri S, Woods WP, van Heerden PV. Air embolism—a case series and review. *Critical Care and Resuscitation*, **6**: 271–6, 2004

http://emedicine.medscape.com/article/761367-diagnosis (accessed 4 March 2010)

Q42 Venous Thromboembolism

a) **List common patient-related risk factors for venous thromboembolism (VTE) (11 marks)**

b) **Outline different methods to prevent perioperative VTE formation (9 marks)**

Aims

It's a trendy topic, new drugs are available, recent NICE guidelines have been published, and hospital morbidity and mortality is still high. This all equals FRCA Examination gold!

a) Common Risk Factors

- Age >60 years
- Continuous long-distance travel prior to or post surgery
- Previous DVT or PE or family history of VTE
- Acute illness requiring critical care admission (e.g. sepsis, respiratory failure)
- Surgery:
  - anaesthetic + surgical time >90mins
  - pelvic or lower limb surgery
  - acute surgical admission with inflammatory or intra-abdominal condition
- Obesity (BMI ≥30kg/m^2)
- Pregnancy
- Dehydration
- Drugs (e.g. oral contraceptive pill, hormone replacement therapy)
- Cancer (± chemo- or radiotherapy)
- Varicose veins with phlebitis
- Immobility (e.g. neurodeficit, prolonged bed-rest, limb in plaster)
- Cardiac disease (e.g. infarction, failure)
- Prolonged presence of a central venous catheter
- Less common: ↓ activated protein C resistance (factor V Leiden mutation), protein C, S and antithrombin deficiencies, antiphospholipid syndrome

b) Thromboprophylaxis

- Thorough assessment of patient to identify high risk
- i) Drugs
  - Stop taking high-risk drugs (e.g. OCP or HRT) 4 weeks prior to surgery
  - Assess risks and benefits of stopping antiplatelet agents
  - Low molecular weight heparin
  - Alternatives (e.g. fondaparinux, dabigatran, rivaroxaban)
  - Unfractionated heparin infusion may be required in patients with mechanical heart valves who normally take warfarin or in renal failure patients
  - Multidisciplinary decision (including GP) as to need for ongoing postoperative VTE thromboprophylaxis
- ii) Mechanical devices
  - Anti-thromboembolic stockings for all surgical patients, except where contraindicated (e.g. peripheral vascular disease, active lower limb infection, neuropathies); single use and measured to fit
  - Foot impulse devices

- Intermittent pneumatic calf or ankle pumps for use perioperatively
- Inferior vena cava filter for patients at very high risk

iii) Other
- Early postoperative physiotherapy to encourage mobility
- Avoid dehydration: administer supplemental IV fluid therapy if required
- Consider the use of regional anaesthesia; evidence to suggest ↓ risk of thromboembolism

Notes

Reference

NICE *Venous Thromboembolism: Reducing the Risk. Quick Reference Guide.* NICE Clinical Guideline 92. London: NICE, 2010

Chapter 2: **Obstetric Anaesthesia**

Q1 Amniotic Fluid Embolism

a) **List the signs and symptoms associated with amniotic fluid embolus (4 marks)**

b) **Discuss the proposed pathogenesis of this syndrome (8 marks)**

c) **Describe the initial management of this scenario (8 marks)**

Aims

Although rare, this is a potentially fatal obstetric emergency. Candidates must be able to treat the clinically deteriorating mother appropriately whilst also being able to describe the possible aetiology. The UK Obstetric Surveillance System (UKOSS) has recently published data regarding incidence and mortality rates, and this makes it likely to appear in an examination at some stage.

a) Signs and Symptoms
   i) Signs
   - Hypoxia and cyanosis
   - Bleeding due to coagulopathy (DIC found in 83%)
   - Cardiovascular collapse
   - Transient hypertension
   - Cardiac arrest
   - Fetal distress (fetal HR <110bpm for >10 minutes or <60bpm for >3 minutes)
   - Pulmonary oedema
   - Seizures: tonic–clonic seen in 50%
   - Uterine atony
   - Bronchospasm
   ii) Symptoms
   - Dyspnoea: often acute onset
   - Cough: may be productive if acute pulmonary oedema
   - Chest pain
   - Headache

b) Pathogenesis
   - Due to the passage of fetal tissue (usually squames, follicles) into the maternal circulation. This requires the presence of:
     - ruptured membranes
     - open maternal veins
     - pressure gradient to drive squames across
   - The systemic reaction to the presence of fetal tissue within the circulation appears to be key. However, the exact process remains elusive
   - Originally it was thought to be a physical consequence similar to a pulmonary embolus. However, later it was proposed to be a two-phase immune response to the antigens contained in fetal tissue.
     - Phase1
       - The response to fetal tissue antigens is the production of vasoactive substances causing pulmonary artery vasospasm resulting in acute right heart failure, hypoxaemia, and hypotension
       - May last up to 30 minutes

◆ Phase 2
 ▪ If the patient survives, the biochemical reaction mediates ↑ capillary permeability, DIC, and uterine atony

c) Management

- Recognition of diagnosis whilst managing the initial consequences
- Structured aggressive resuscitation required quickly to reduce mortality
- Call for help: anaesthetic assistance and obstetric/midwife assistance for the fetus
- Airway: consider intubating if obstructed and profoundly hypoxic
- Breathing: administer high-flow oxygen and CPAP initially to treat hypoxia, increase intra-alveolar pressure, and reduce pulmonary oedema. Ultimately, invasive ventilation with PEEP may be required
- Circulation: treat hypotension with fluids and vasopressors to maintain systemic organ perfusion. Invasive monitoring and large-bore IV access are established to provide fluid resuscitation and monitor cardiovascular status
- Left lateral tilt in pregnant women: reduces aortocaval compression and improves blood pressure and placental perfusion
- Haemorrhage
  ◆ DIC usually from activation of tissue factor and factor X
  ◆ Send bloods for FBC, clotting, and fibrinogen; activate major haemorrhage protocol
  ◆ Involve haematology clinicians early: blood product requirements as guided by results (factor VIIa has been used in this setting)
  ◆ Consider TEG analysis if available
- Uterine atony: obstetric involvement and oxytocic agents, including compression and massage, will help ↑ tone and may aid in reducing blood loss
- Seizures: termination with short-acting anticonvulsants (e.g. benzodiazepines)
- Fetus: delivery via Caesarean section is warranted if circulatory arrest persists for >5 minutes

Notes

....

....

....

....

....

....

References

Dedhia JD, Mushambi MC. Amniotic fluid embolism. *Continuing Education in Anaesthesia, Critical Care & Pain*, **7**, 152–6, 2007

Gist RS, Stafford IP, Leibowitz AB, Beilin Y. Amniotic fluid embolism. *Anesthesia and Analgesia* **108**: 1599–1602, 2009

Knight MD, Tuffnell D, Brocklehurst P, *et al.*. Incidence and risk factors for amniotic-fluid embolism. *Obstetrics and Gynecology*, **115**: 910–17, 2010

https://www.npeu.ox.ac.uk/ukoss/current-surveillance/amf (accessed 9 September 2010)

Q2 Saving Mothers' Lives

a) **List the most common causes of direct maternal death in the UK (4 marks)**

b) **Outline risk factors which increase the likelihood of maternal mortality (6 marks)**

c) **What anaesthetic-related recommendations exist to improve perinatal maternal safety? (10 marks)**

Aims

This is a very topical question which has appeared in recent settings of the SAQ paper. It is triennial so is likely to make an appearance in the examination again soon.

a) Direct Maternal Death (Saving Mothers' Lives 2003-2005)

- Thromboembolic disease
- Pre-eclampsia or eclampsia
- Haemorrhage
- Early pregnancy complications (e.g. ectopic, spontaneous miscarriage, termination)
- Genital tract sepsis or trauma
- Anaesthetic-related causes

b) Risk Factors

- Older mothers: ↑ incidence of comorbidities (e.g. cardiac disease)
- Improvements in cardiac surgery leading to increased survival of congenital heart disease patients to child-bearing age
- ↑ incidence of assisted conception leads to complications of multiple pregnancies
- Obesity
- Lifestyle (e.g. smoking, drinking, substance abuse, domestic abuse)
- Immigration (communication barriers, poorer health or undiagnosed medical conditions, ↑ incidence of TB, HIV/AIDS)
- Poverty, unemployment, lack of education
- Lack of prenatal counselling
- Psychiatric disease

c) Recommendations

i) Prenatal anaesthetic assessment for high-risk women (multidisciplinary approach)
   - Obesity (BMI >30kg/m^2), cardiac disease, epilepsy, diabetes, autoimmune disease
   - Dedicated preassessment clinic for history, examination of CVS, respiratory, airway, back
   - Perinatal anaesthetic plan: discussion of risks, regional techniques

ii) Involvement with Obstetric Care of High-Risk Patients
   - Clinical advice and support for mothers with pregnancy-induced hypertension or pre-eclampsia and an active involvement in the delivery plan
   - Awareness of placental location in high-risk mothers (e.g. placenta praevia with previous Caesarean section and the potential risk of haemorrhage)
   - Identification of pregnant patients at high risk of thromboembolic disease and initiation of appropriate thromboprophylaxis

iii) The unwell parturient
- To provide teaching and training to delivery suite staff in Advanced Life Support and the recognition and management of unwell pregnant patients
- Presence of an early warning obstetric scoring system for detection and prevention of clinical deterioration, with appropriate clinical referral to anaesthetist or intensivist
- Active clinical leadership in early recognition of the unwell pregnant patient and initiating management plan to prevent maternal collapse (e.g. sepsis or haemorrhage)

iv) Guidelines for:
- Treatment of the obese pregnant woman
- Treatment of sepsis in pregnancy
- Major obstetric haemorrhage protocol
- Failed intubation in the obstetric patient
- Epidural device drug delivery (prevents wrong-route delivery)

v) Senior Involvement
- Trainee anaesthetists to recognize and accept their limits of clinical competence
- Direct access 24 hours a day to consultant for advice and help with high-risk cases
- Senior anaesthetic input to be available for management of morbidly obese parturients

Notes

- *Direct deaths*: deaths resulting from obstetric complications of the pregnant state (pregnancy, labour, and puerperium), interventions, omissions, incorrect treatment, or a chain of events resulting from any of the above
- *Indirect deaths*: deaths resulting from previous existing disease, or disease that developed during pregnancy and which was not due to direct obstetric causes, but which was aggravated by the physiological effects of pregnancy
- *Coincidental deaths*: deaths from unrelated causes which happen to occur in pregnancy or the puerperium

References

Lewis G (ed). *The Confidential Enquiry into Maternal and Child Health (CEMACH). Saving Mothers' Lives: Reviewing Maternal Deaths to Make Motherhood Safer 2003-2005. Seventh Report on Confidential Enquiries into Maternal Deaths in the United Kingdom.* London: CEMACH, 2007

OAA/AAGBI Guidelines for Obstetric Anaesthetic Services (revised) London: OSA, AAGBI, 2005

Q3 Epidural Drug Delivery

a) **List the potential critical incidents that can occur with drug delivery via the epidural route (7 marks)**

b) **How can organizations prevent or minimize epidural drug delivery incidents? (13 marks)**

Aims

Extensive media coverage has highlighted the fatal effects of wrong drug delivery via the epidural route. Topical subjects such as this have a high chance of appearance in the Final FRCA examination in some guise, so are well worth reading and understanding.

a) Critical Incidents

- Epidural drug delivered via wrong route (e.g. IV, IM, or even intrathecal)
- IV or IM drug delivered via epidural route
- Wrong epidural drug (e.g. lidocaine instead of bupivacaine)
- Incorrect dose of epidural drug delivered (e.g. volume and concentration)
- Drug dose, concentration, delivery method incorrectly documented in notes
- Epidural delivery device incorrectly primed, set up, programmed, or used
- Missed doses of epidural drug
- Error in drug supply (e.g. boxes or vials incorrectly labelled)
- Use of expired epidural drug
- Epidural drug not stored correctly (e.g. bupivacaine–fentanyl mix should be in a locked controlled-drug cupboard)

b) Prevention or Minimization of Incidents

i) Labelling
- Clear labelling on packaging, infusion bags, and syringes: FOR EPIDURAL USE ONLY
- Use different coloured and designed bags, syringes, and infusion lines (e.g. yellow) to distinguish from IV drugs
- Suggested incompatibility between epidural bags and IV infusion giving sets

ii) Doses and Concentrations
- Limit the range of doses or concentrations available for epidural route administration to avoid potential dose errors
- Ensure that epidural doses, concentrations, and infusions are checked by a second qualified person prior to administration
- Regular annual audit of epidural administration should be practised to ensure adherence to national and local guidelines
- Minimize complicated epidural drug preparation by providing ready-mixed bags (e.g. 0.125% bupivacaine with 2mcg/mL fentanyl in a 500mL bag)

iii) Storage
- Store all epidural drug syringes, bags, and infusions separately from IV drugs
- Confirm that the pharmacy is sending the correct epidural drug to the correct clinical area (e.g. syringes vs. infusion bags)

iv) Administration Sets
- Use designated epidural giving sets which may be identified clearly with labelling (e.g. EPIDURAL) and a colour (e.g. yellow line)

- Ensure clear procedures are present to guide clinicians in the correct set-up and labelling of epidural drug administration

v) Epidural Delivery Devices
  - These delivery devices must be clearly labelled FOR EPIDURAL USE ONLY so that they are clearly distinguishable from IV delivery devices which may also be present in the same clinical area (e.g. syntocinon infusion in maternity)
  - These should be standardized for epidural delivery with preset codes and epidural drug protocols relevant to that clinical area

vi) Staff training
  - All staff involved in the preparation, administration, and clinical care of patients receiving epidural drugs should undergo formal training in epidural drug preparation, delivery, and monitoring
  - For inexperienced staff, there should be competencies to sign off and supervision by senior staff before solo supervision of patients with epidural drug delivery is allowed
  - Staff should be trained in the recognition and management of local anaesthetic toxicity

Notes

Reference

National Patient Safety Agency. *Epidural Injections and Infusions 2007.* http://www.nrls.npsa.nhs.uk/resources/?entryid45=59807 (Accessed 8 November 2009)

Q4 General Anaesthesia for Caesarean Section

a) **List the indications for Caesarean section under general anaesthesia (6 marks)**

b) **Outline the preoperative preparation and management of anaesthetic induction in a woman requiring an emergency Caesarean section for fetal bradycardia (14 marks)**

Aims

Provision of a GA Caesarean section is fundamental to the practice of obstetric anaesthesia. All trainees must demonstrate competency and understanding of the process prior to on-call duties, and this must be conveyed in your answer even if you have not performed large numbers of Caesarean sections when you sit the examination.

a) Indications for GA

- Urgency of Caesarean section: either maternal or fetal risk of morbidity or mortality
- Failure or inability to perform regional technique (e.g. spinal abnormalities, morbid obesity)
- Failure of regional anaesthesia to provide adequate blockade
- Contraindication to performing regional technique (e.g. maternal refusal, coagulopathic, thrombocytopenic, local or systemic sepsis)
- Severely compromised or altered maternal cardiovascular physiology (e.g. haemorrhage or cardiac disease)
- In elective or semi-elective cases with a high risk of haemorrhage (e.g. placental implantation syndromes)

b) GA Caesarean Section

- It is assumed that anaesthetic equipment and drugs have been checked

i) Pre-assessment
  - May have minimal time; therefore need to be concise
  - Past anaesthetic history, family history of anaesthetic problems
  - Past medical history, drug history, allergies
  - Last food and drink
  - Airway assessment
  - Consent: RSI technique, cricoid pressure, sore throat, dental damage, postoperative analgesia myalgia
  - Commence *in utero* resuscitation: ensure left lateral tilt, administer IV fluids and O_2, stop syntocinon infusion if running, and consider tocolysis

ii) In Theatre
  - Reattach CTG machine and check whether there is time to perform a regional technique
  - Full AAGBI monitoring is attached; induction is on the operating table
  - One or more wide-bore cannulas is inserted or checked for patency; FBC, U&E, clotting, and cross-match samples are taken
  - Ensure left lateral tilt or wedge on operating theatre to prevent aortocaval compression
  - Antacid prophylaxis: IV ranitidine 50mg and metoclopramide 10mg; PO sodium citrate 30mL 0.3M

- The bladder is catheterized, the skin draped and prepared, and the surgeon scrubbed and ready to operate prior to induction

iii) Induction
- Pre-oxygenation in the head-up position: 100% O_2 via a tight-fitting mask for ≥3 minutes or 4–5 vital capacity breaths
- Thiopentone 5mg/kg lean body weight rapidly followed by suxamethonium 1.5mg/kg with simultaneous cricoid pressure as consciousness is lost
- Intubation of trachea and confirm placement with capnography, bilateral chest expansion, and auscultation.
- Maintain anaesthesia and muscle relaxation with O_2, N_2O, or air, a volatile agent, and NDMB
- Important to consider the additional use of opiates (e.g. alfentanil) with induction agents to obtund the laryngoscopy pressor effect in pre-eclampsia or cardiac disease. The paediatrician must be informed

Notes

Reference

McGlennan A, Mustafa A. General anaesthesia for Caesarean section. *Continuing Education in Anaesthesia, Critical Care & Pain*, **9**, 148–51, 2009

Q5 HELLP Syndrome

a) **Define HELLP syndrome (4 marks)**

b) **Outline clinical features and laboratory findings associated with HELLP syndrome (6 marks)**

c) **What is your management of this disease? (10 marks)**

Aims

This is an important and relatively common situation. You must be able to clearly demonstrate an understanding of when this complication of pre-eclampsia will exclude regional anaesthesia, as well as recognizing this important sign of a potential obstetric emergency and its management.

a) Definition

- **H**aemolysis, **E**levated **L**iver enzymes, **L**ow **P**latelets
- Severe complication of pre-eclampsia
- Maternal mortality ~1%, high fetal mortality (2° to premature delivery)
- Presentation: 80% antenatal (majority before 36/40) and 20% postnatal

b) Clinical Features and Laboratory Investigations

- Generalized malaise, viral symptoms, nausea and vomiting
- Right upper quadrant tenderness, peripheral oedema, weight gain. NB: Hypertension and proteinuria are *not* prerequisites for diagnosis
- Platelet count <100 × 10^9/L
- Hepatic function deterioration: deranged clotting, ↓ albumin, ↑ AST and ALT
- Evidence of haemolysis: ↑ bilirubin and LDH, evidence of haemolysis on blood smear

c) Management Aims

- HDU or ICU care once diagnosed
- Thorough explanation and counselling re risks and delivery
- Usually a planned early delivery before clinical deterioration occurs
- Some evidence to suggest that high-dose steroids are of benefit: ↑ platelet count, ↑ birth-weight

i) Fluid Balance
   - Principle aim: avoid pulmonary oedema 2° to fluid overload whilst maintaining perfusion to vital organs (including antenatal placental perfusion)
   - May be challenging, because:
     - higher risk of perinatal haemorrhage requiring fluid resuscitation and/or blood products
     - leaky capillaries (2° to systemic vasoconstriction and inflammatory cascade) promoting ↑ tissue oedema
     - deranged hepatic function promoting coagulopathy and exacerbating any haemorrhage
   - Early renal replacement therapy considered to avert pulmonary oedema formation and the need for intubation and mechanical ventilation
   - Convulsions are treated as for pre-eclampsia (i.e Mg^{2+} therapy) whilst ruling out other organic causes

Notes

Reference

Dresner M. HELLP syndrome. In: Waldmann C, Soni N, Rhodes A, eds. *Oxford Desk Reference: Critical Care*. Oxford University Press, 2008; 522–3

Q6 Labour Pain Pathways

a) Describe the different pain pathways during labour (9 marks)

b) List the indications for providing regional analgesia in labour (11 marks)

Aims

An understanding of obstetric analgesic requirements is necessary to provide a satisfactory anaesthetic service on the labour ward. An anatomical approach of how to provide this acts as a good framework with which to tackle the problem, especially when primary techniques fail.

a) Pain Pathways in Labour

- Comprises uterine and extra-uterine pathways
- i) First Stage
  - Pain source is from both uterine and extra-uterine sources, i.e. cervical dilation and uterine contraction.
  - Impulses are transmitted via uterine sympathetic axons in T10–12 located in the superior and inferior hypogastric plexuses, with some minor input via vessels in the tubo-ovarian ligament.
  - Displacement of other abdominal viscera by the gravid uterus can also manifest during labour, and are mainly transmitted via the coeliac plexus. The diaphragm receives its sensory innervation via the phrenic nerve

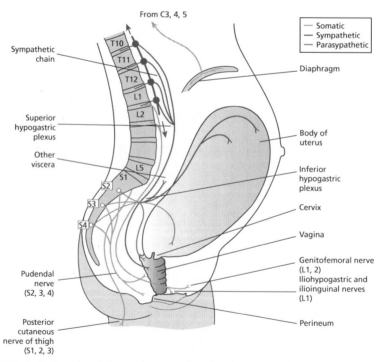

Figure 8. Peripheral pain pathways during labour

ii) Second Stage
- Extra-uterine pain is mainly vaginal and perineal in origin, with impulses conveyed via the pudendal nerve (S2–4), with variable input from the genitofemoral nerve (L1–2)
- Extra-uterine compression of adjacent structures is often related to fetal position (i.e. occipito-posterior lie) and causes compression of adjacent viscera, usually with associated low backache. These impulses are usually transmitted via L5–S1

b) Indications for Regional Analgesia in Labour

i) Maternal
- Non-obstetric surgery: allows avoidance of GA, although non-essential surgery is best postponed until the post-partum period
- Obstetric surgery, i.e. elective Caesarean section, repair of delivery tears, manual removal of placenta
- Pre-eclampsia: ↑ placental blood flow and reduction of circulating catecholamines
- Cardiac disease
  - Regurgitant valve lesions benefit from reduction in afterload and promotion of forward flow
  - Stenotic lesions need extreme caution to maintain adequate SVR
- Respiratory disease
  - Optimize ventilation in patients with reduced ventilatory capacity. Caution with high block and loss of intercostal accessory muscle input
- Obesity
  - ↑ incidence of prolonged labour, comorbid maternal disease, and postoperative complications in this cohort makes regional anaesthesia desirable
- Central nervous system
  - Prevention of large swings in ICP in patients with abnormal anatomy, i.e. Arnold–Chiari malformations.
  - Spinal cord injury patients have high probability of developing autonomic dysreflexia during labour contractions. A good regional block can obtund or block this pathway.

ii) Labour
- Maternal request
- Labour analgesia: epidural, combined spinal–epidural, pudendal block
- Labour with potential complications
  - Multiple gestation pregnancy
  - Malpresentation, i.e. breech
  - Induction or augmentation of labour
  - Anticipated long labour, i.e. primiparous women

iii) Fetal
- For babies at high risk of complications
- Promotes placental blood flow '(especially important in severe preeclampsia)

Notes

....

....

....

....

....

....

Q7 Major Obstetric Haemorrhage

You are called to see a 26-year-old woman who is bleeding 2 hours post normal vaginal delivery. She is listed for an urgent examination under anaesthesia.

a) **Describe your initial assessment of this patient (7 marks)**

b) **What are i) the surgical (6 marks) and ii) the non-surgical (7 marks) methods of treating a major obstetric haemorrhage?**

Aims

This combines multiple issues, including management of a major haemorrhage, a potentially difficult airway in term women, and an approach to a potentially unstable patient. Your answer must include all the key points, whilst giving the impression of familiarity with this scenario to convey confidence in managing these patients.

a) Initial Assessment

- Airway: if not patent or obstructed, attempt to relieve obstruction with basic airway manoeuvres. If unsuccessful, prepare to intubate and ventilate
- Breathing: administer 100% O_2 via a non-rebreathe mask, measure respiratory rate and pulse oximetry, auscultate the lungs, and perform an ABG (if time)
- Circulation
  - Ensure ×2 wide-bore venous cannulae and take blood for FBC, U&E, clotting (including fibrinogen) and a cross-match sample
  - Measure HR, NIBP, capillary refill time; commence IV fluids and insert a urinary catheter
  - Consider O −ve blood transfusion if cross-matched blood is delayed
- Disability: assess GCS; if <8/15, intubation and ventilation is warranted
- History: previous anaesthetics, family history of of anaesthetic problems, comorbidities, drug history, allergies, airway assessment, last food and drink
- Investigations: most recent blood results

b) Methods of Treating Haemorrhage

i) Surgical
- Vigorous bimanual uterine massage
- Aortic compression
- Manual removal of retained placenta
- Repair of ruptured uterus, or lacerated vaginal wall or cervix
- Laparotomy and uterine compression (with uterine replacement if inversion)
- Haemostatic uterine suturing (B-Lynch)
- Tamponade balloon insertion
- Bilateral ligation of uterine or internal iliac arteries
- Hysterectomy

ii) Non-Surgical Methods
- IV syntocinon 5–10IU bolus slowly ± infusion of 30–40IU syntocinon in 500mL 0.9% saline at 100–125mL/hour. Be aware: bolus can cause hypotension and tachycardia
- IV or IM ergometrine 250–500mcg: can cause nausea, vomiting, and hypertension. Should be avoided in pre-eclamptic patients
- IM 15-methylprostoglandin $F_{2\alpha}$ (Hemabate™) 0.25–0.5mg (15min intervals up to a maximum of five doses)

- PR misoprostol 800–1000mcg
- Packed red cells: improve Hb concentration (may require O –ve blood)
- Fresh frozen plasma: if PT/APTT >1.5
- Platelets: if platelet count <50 × 10^9/L
- Cryoprecipitate: if fibrinogen <0.5g/L
- IV recombinant factor VIIa (NovoSeven®) 100mcg/kg: consider if corrected PT, APTT, platelets, fibrinogen, pH >7.2, core body temperature > 36°C
- Calcium replacement: due to citrate chelation in massive blood transfusion
- Antifibrinolytics (e.g. tranexamic acid 1g IV)
- Radiological: uterine artery embolization

Notes

Q8 Multiple Gestation Pregnancy

A 32-year-old woman pregnant with twins has arrived on the delivery suite complaining of regular 'tightenings'.

a) List the potential complications associated with a multiple gestation birth (10 marks)

b) Outline the anaesthetic management of this woman, including relevant analgesic options (10 marks)

Aims

This question has appeared before in the SAQ paper and is a scenario which most anaesthetists will have been involved in at some point in their careers. Your answer should convey an appreciation of the additional risks and logistical issues whilst not forgetting the classic of when to give the oxytocics.

a) Complications

i) Maternal Complications
- Preterm labour
- Premature rupture of membranes
- Pre-eclampsia and eclampsia
- Antepartum haemorrhage
- Placental abruption
- Prolonged labour
- Uterine atony
- Trauma to obstetric organs
- Higher chance of an instrumental or Caesarean section delivery
- Postpartum haemorrhage
- Increased weight gain (may complicate airway management)
- $\downarrow$ TLC and FRC (quicker to desaturate during apnoea post induction of anaesthesia)
- $\uparrow$ gravid uterus further compromises oesophageal sphincters ($\uparrow$ risk of regurgitation and aspiration)
- $\uparrow$ fetal weights and volume of amniotic fluid

ii) Fetal Complications
- Congenital abnormalities
- Intrauterine growth restriction and death
- Malpresentation (especially of second twin following delivery of first twin)
- Twin–twin transfusion syndrome
- Preterm delivery
- Polyhydramnios
- Umbilical cord prolapsed
- Umbilical cord entanglement

b) Anaesthetic Management

- Early antenatal anaesthetic assessment, explaining relevant risks outlined above
- Standard obstetric anaesthetic history and examination to include airway, back, and veins
- Explain $\uparrow$ risk of instrumental or Caesarean section delivery. Therefore analgesia options should be discussed

- Early epidural in labour is the ideal analgesia for both labour pains and delivery if an instrumental or Caesarean section delivery is required
- Ensure wide-bore cannulation (×2 if considered very high risk for bleeding) and blood tests: FBC, U&E, clotting, and cross-match sample
- Regular ranitidine ± metoclopramide in labour
- Ensure vigilance in managing the epidural: low threshold for resite if not adequate analgesia
- Regular communication with obstetricians regarding progress of labour and delivery plans
- Ideally, delivery should be in theatre to allow quick progression to instrumentation or Caesarean section if required
- Patient should always be in the left lateral tilt or full left lateral position to minimize risk of aortocaval compression (*never* left supine)
- Early 'top-up' of epidural analgesia will facilitate instrumental delivery (especially if malpresentation of the second twin requires delivery by Caesarean section following vaginal delivery of the first twin)

Notes

Q9 Non-Obstetric Surgery in Pregnancy

A 27-year-old woman, who is currently 26 weeks pregnant, is listed for an emergency appendicectomy.

a) List the potential complications of anaesthesia unique to this case (10 marks)

b) Describe anaesthetic options for the management of this patient (10 marks)

Aims

This is a great topic for the SAQ section as it tests the candidate's knowledge of early obstetric anaesthetic management for a normally straightforward anaesthetic emergency. Many hospitals have a pro forma which will act as an alternative template to the answer set out below.

a) Complications

i) Maternal

The consequences of pregnancy have modified maternal physiology significantly. Her response to GA will be different in all her organ systems as listed below.

- Central nervous system
  - ↑ sensitivity to opiates and volatile anaesthetic agents
  - ↑ probability of delayed recovery
- Respiratory
  - Displacement of diaphragm resulting in ↓ FRC, coupled with ↑ O_2 consumption results in faster desaturation on induction of GA
  - ↑ incidence of difficult or failed intubation in pregnant women compared with non-obstetric population
- Gastrointestinal
  - ↑ probability of aspiration following relaxation of lower oesophageal sphincter and delayed gastric emptying (pain, opiates exacerbate this further)
- Cardiovascular system
  - Aortocaval compression may cause significant ↓ in venous return and subsequent hypotension.
- Musculoskeletal
  - ↑ ligament laxity due to higher progesterone levels increases the probability of joint hyperextension during surgery
- Haematological
  - ↑ levels of clotting factors elevates the risk of peri- and postoperative thrombosis

ii) Fetal

- Miscarrriage: levels ↑ from 1.4% to 5.9% in the second trimester (no discrimination between site of surgery and elevation in risk)
- Premature labour
  - ↑ risk is seen after 22/40
  - More risk with abdominal and pelvic surgery

b) Anaesthetic Options

- If at all possible, postpone all elective surgery during pregnancy until after delivery
- Perform the operation on a site with obstetric services, and ensure that they are aware of the patient. Consider peri-operative fetal heart rate monitoring and CTG tracing with a midwife or obstetrician who is trained to interpret it

- Discuss the risk of premature labour with the patient, as detailed, and ensure that she is aware of the risks involved.
- Consult the obstetric team regarding the use of steroids for fetal maturation
- Ensure senior surgical and anaesthetic team members are involved to minimize duration of surgery
- Be aware of which drugs are safe to use in pregnancy (avoid NSAIDs)
- If there is concern regarding the airway and an awake fibreoptic induction is planned, avoid the use of cocaine for topical anaesthesia of the nose – oral route is preferred
- RSI is indicated
- Woman is positioned in left lateral tilt to ↓ aortocaval compression
- Avoid using the nose for temperature monitoring or gastric decompression (high risk of epistaxis due to vessel congestion/engorgement)
- Ventilate to normal $EtCO_2$ for pregnancy (4kPa) by ↑ TV not RR; consider PEEP
- Aim to maintain placental perfusion with strict BP control perioperatively
- If laparascopic surgery is planned:
  - consider an arterial line to allow accurate monitoring of BP and $Pa\,CO_2$
  - limit pressure within the pneumoperitoneum to <15mmHg
- Ensure perioperative prophylactic prevention of venous thromboembolism with calf compressors and compression stockings. Postoperative prevention with hydration, physiotherapy, and anticoagulation is essential

Notes

Q10 **Obesity in Obstetrics**

You are asked to review a 41-year-old primiparous women whose booking BMI was 44kg/m² and is now 36 weeks pregnant.

a) **List the complications posed by obesity in pregnancy (9 marks)**

b) **What advice would you give regarding analgesia for labour and delivery? (11 marks)**

Aims

Obstetric obesity is a highly topical subject which continues to provide challenges for anaesthetists and which has and will continue to feature in the FRCA examination.

a) Complications

i) Antenatal
   - ↑ risk of comorbidities (e.g. gestational diabetes, pregnancy-induced hypertension, pre-eclampsia, venous thromboembolic disease)

ii) Perinatal
   - ↑ incidence of instrumental and Caesarean section delivery
   - Difficulty in IV access
   - Difficult to site RA techniques because of poor anatomical landmarks
   - Higher risk of unilateral, failed, or even high regional block because of altered spread of local anaesthetic secondary to fat compression of the epidural space
   - Difficulty in estimating lean body weight to calculate drug doses
   - ↑ incidence of reflux and difficult or failed intubation should GA be required
   - Risk to staff involved in mobilizing patients post RA or GA delivery
   - Equipment issues, i.e. maximum weight supported by delivery bed and operating table

iii) Postnatal
   - ↑ incidence of postoperative infection (e.g. surgical wound or chest infection)
   - ↑ incidence of thromboembolic disorders, i.e. DVT or PE
   - ↑ incidence of cardiorespiratory complications (e.g. pulmonary oedema, postpartum cardiomyopathy, postoperative hypoxia, ↑ O_2 requirements)

b) Analgesic Management
   - Need to emphasize ↑ risk of abnormal labour and difficulty in siting epidural
   - Advantages of epidural in labour (e.g. analgesia, easier to tolerate tocolytics, ↓ risk of DVT)
   - Emphasis on siting epidural early to allow for difficult insertion
   - Examination of the back at the same time may identify difficult anatomy
   - Potential avoidance of GA
   - Options should epidural fail to be sited (i.e. remifentanil PCA) and assess for difficult airway
   - Complications of epidurals (e.g. hypotension, motor block) and possible effects on labour (e.g. relative ↑ in instrumental delivery)
   - Discussion should focus on options of GA vs. RA and relative benefits of RA (i.e. avoidance of complications of GA, aspiration, difficult or failed intubation, hypoxia)
   - ↑ risk of effects of GA on fetus and requirement for neonatal intervention and resuscitation
   - Regional technique should be discussed, including complications and side effects

- Consider a combined spinal–epidural (CSE) for added benefit of manipulating the block for Caesarean section as dermatomes are often difficult to assess in morbidly obese patients and the duration of surgery is often longer
- Discuss method of ensuring adequate block and management of pain of discomfort:
  - epidural top-up if CSE used
  - IV bolus on fentanyl, especially if post-delivery
  - Entonox via face mask
- Possible conversion to GA if unable to produce adequate block once surgery commenced
- Touch and pressure sensations during surgery are normal in a working regional block

Notes

References

Francis S, May A. Pregnant women with significant medical conditions: anaesthetic implications. *Continuing Education in Anaesthesia, Critical Care & Pain,* **4**: 95–7, 2004

http://www.aagbi.org/publications/guidelines/docs/Obesity07.pdf (accessed 25 May 2010)

Q11 **Obstetric Consent**

A 24-year-old primiparous women is requesting an epidural for labour analgesia.

a) Define consent (3 marks)

b) What problems exist in consenting obstetric patients for an epidural? (6 marks)

c) Describe how you would consent this women for an epidural, including the risks of the procedure (11 marks)

Aims

Informed consent in labour has always been a controversial area. Candidates must be aware of the process of obstetric consent and be able to list all the major risks of performing an epidural.

a) Consent

- Permission for a treatment, investigation, or physical contact with a patient
- To be valid, consent must be given voluntarily by an appropriately informed person
- The patient must have capacity, i.e. the ability to understand the consequences, weigh up the benefits and risks, and retain information relevant to the decision-making process

b) Obstetric Problems

- Controversy over the judgement and capacity of a labouring woman
  - Considerable physical and psychological stress
  - Pain
  - Fatigue
  - Anxiety
  - Drugs (e.g. Entonox, opiates)
- There may be obstetric or anaesthetic reasons for the procedure which the patient may not comprehend (e.g. pre-eclampsia, obesity)
- In some cases, it is a procedure with risk of severe complications in a young fit person

c) Consent

- Introduction to woman and partner to establish rapport
- Concise and relevant anaesthetic and obstetric history to ensure no contraindications to procedure
- Check blood results to ensure that coagulopathy or thrombocytopenia is not present
- Explain how the procedure is performed and what is required of the woman, i.e. position, minimal movement, signalling of contractions
- Explain benefits of procedure
  - Superior analgesia
  - Rest
  - Provision of syntocinon
  - Ability to 'top-up' for surgical anaesthesia
  - Lowering of BP in pre-eclampsia
- Explain risks of procedure (controversy as to what should be included re rarer risks— decided on individual basis):
  - Inadequate or unilateral block, failure and potential for resite of epidural
  - Bruising to back at site of injection

- Itching, shivering, urinary retention, motor block (1 in 10 chance of each symptom)
- Headache (should quote personal figures): 1 in 100–150
- Hypotension (easily treated with fluids and drugs)
- Temporary nerve damage: 1 in 3000-7000
- Intravascular injection, total spinal: 1 in 10,000
- Persistent or permanent nerve damage: 1 in 25,000–160,000
- Meningitis: 1 in 100,000–1,000,000
- Paralysis: <1 in 100,000

Notes

_____

_____

_____

_____

_____

_____

_____

_____

_____

_____

_____

References

Baker B, Jenkins K. Anaesthetic risk. In: Allman KG, Wilson I, eds. *Oxford Handbook of Anaesthesia* (2nd edn). Oxford University Press, 2006; 19–21

Kelly GD, Blunt C, Moore PA, Lewis M. (2004). Consent for regional anaesthesia in the United Kingdom: what is material risk? *International Journal of Obstetric Anesthesia*, **13**: 71–4, 2004

National Audit of Major Complications of Central Neuraxial Block in the United Kingdom. 3rd National Audit Project. London: Royal College of Anaesthetists, 2009

Q12 Post-Dural Puncture Headache

You are inserting an epidural for labour analgesia. Upon achieving loss of resistance to saline, you remove the stylet and witness a jet of clear fluid pouring from the Tuohy needle.

a) Outline your subsequent management during the procedure (7 marks)

b) List the risk factors for dural puncture and post-dural puncture headache (PDPH) in obstetrics (6 marks)

c) Outline the management of a patient who has developed a headache 48 hours post dural puncture (7 marks)

Aims

Immediate intervention is required when PDPH is encountered. Most complaints regarding this procedure usually stem from poor management of the headache rather than the fact that it has occurred. Your answer will need to demonstrate a familiarity with treating the headache and the emphasis on communication required to ensure that patients and relatives feel informed of the likely course of events.

a) Management During Epidural Insertion

- Inform patient of occurrence of dural puncture
- i) Analgesic options
  - Site spinal catheter for labour analgesia:
    - anaesthetist-only 'top-up'
    - low-volume LA to be administered according to spinal catheter protocol
    - warn patient of increased probability of motor block and hypotension
    - slight ↓ in incidence of headache if catheter threaded as though to elicit fibrotic reaction at puncture site (controversial as evidence is weak)
    - once pain controlled, discuss management (i.e. headache, follow-up)
    - discuss with obstetric team and consultant anaesthetist on call
  - Attempt to resite epidural in same site, or
  - Attempt to resite epidural in different site, usually a space higher as there is potential to thread the new catheter through the hole in the dura
  - Abandon the procedure and use an alternative analgesia regimen, i.e. remifentanil PCA

b) Risk Factors for Dural Puncture and Postdural Puncture Headache

- i) Dural Puncture
  - Technically difficult procedure, e.g. moving patient, poor position
  - Abnormal anatomy i.e. scoliosis
  - Multiple attempts
  - Insertion during contractions
  - Experience of the operator
  - Loss of resistance to air
  - Previous dural puncture
  - High BMI
- ii) Postdural Puncture Headache
  - Previous history of headaches postpartum
  - Low BMI

- Large-diameter needle
- Cutting needle
- Multiple attempts
- Dehydration
- Bed-rest
- Perpendicular needle alignment

c) Management of a Headache 2 Days Postpartum

- Full history and examination to determine likely aetiology of the headache, including:
  - postural elements
  - pattern through the day
  - aggravating or relieving factors
  - previous history of headaches and presence of comorbidities
  - relief of the headache with abdominal pressure or straining
- Exclude overt neurological signs; if concerned refer to neurology for assessment
- Once a diagnosis of PDPH is made management is as follows.

i) Conservative
  - Bed-rest reduces severity of pain but will not aid resolution of the symptoms
  - Abdominal binders are not routinely used in clinical practice

ii) Pharmacological
  - Fluids (PO or IV)
  - Analgesia: paracetamol, NSAIDs, codeine, strong opiates PRN
  - Evidence for the use of atypical therapies (e.g. cerebral vasoconstrictors) is weak:
    - caffeine (800–1000mg/day = 8–10 cups coffee daily)
    - $5\text{-}HT_1$ anatagonists (i.e. sumitriptan)
    - Theophylline
    - Methergine, a novel vasoconstrictor with a few case reports documenting some success
  - ↑ CSF production: ACTH (1.5mcg/kg)

iii) Interventional
  - Epidural blood patch (5–25 ml) ± epidural opiates
    - Patient lies flat for minimum of 2 hours post procedure to aid clot formation. Therefore advise to go to toilet before procedure.
    - Patients classically report instant relief of headache
    - Serial blood patches are associated with ↑ rates of success
    - If >2 blood patches: consider referral to neurology for further assessment
    - Contraindicated if signs of concurrent infection
  - Epidural saline bolus (if contraindication to blood-patching, range volume 30–60mL) or infusion (1L over 24 hours)

Notes

....

....

....

....

....

....

....

....

....

....

....

Reference

Turnbull, DK, Shepherd DB. Post-dural puncture headache: pathogenesis, prevention and treatment. *British Journal of Anaesthesia*, **91**: 718–29, 2003

Q13 Venothromboembolism and Pregnancy

a) **List the peripartum risk factors for venous thromboembolic (VTE) disease during pregnancy (8 marks)**

b) **Discuss the antenatal assessment and management of pregnant women at high risk of VTE (5 marks)**

c) **What are the recommendations for thromboprophylaxis in all women following delivery? (7 marks)**

Aims

Currently, more women on the labour ward are at increased risk of VTE due to comorbidities, obesity, etc. Different formulations of anticoagulation and timing of administration have a direct impact on administrating neuraxial procedures. A significant proportion of women still suffer from peripheral and central venous thrombosis, and clinical awareness is essential.

a) Risk Factors

i) Pre-existing
- Previous venous thromboembolism
- Thrombophilia (e.g. antithrombin deficiency, protein C or S deficiency, factor V Leiden mutation, antiphospholipid syndrome)
- Medical comorbidities (e.g. CVS/respiratory disease, SLE, cancer, inflammatory bowel disease, nephrotic syndrome, sickle cell disease, IV drug abuser)
- Age >35 years
- Obesity (BMI >30kg/m²)
- Family history of VTE
- Smoking
- Significant varicose veins (symptomatic/associated phlebitis or skin changes)
- Paraplegia

ii) Obstetric
- Multiple gestation pregnancies, assisted reproductive techniques (e.g. IVF)
- Multiparous woman
- Pre-eclampsia
- Peripartum surgical procedure (e.g. appendicectomy, laparoscopic cholecystectomy)
- Prolonged labour
- Forceps delivery
- Caesarean section
- Postpartum haemorrhage

iii) Reversible Causes
- Hyperemesis and/or dehydration
- Ovarian hyperstimulation syndrome
- Admission or immobility (≥ 3days bed-rest) (e.g. symphysis pubis dysfunction)
- Systemic infection (requiring antibiotics or admission to hospital) (e.g. pneumonia, postpartum wound infection)
- Long-distance travel (>4 hours)

b) Antenatal Assessment and Management

- Pre-pregnancy counselling with a prospective management plan for thromboprophylaxis during pregnancy. For example, a referral should be made to a consultant obstetrician or a clinical expert in thrombosis in pregnancy
- If previous history of VTE, women should be tested for thrombophilia
- Antenatal thromboprophylaxis should begin as early in pregnancy as possible
- Low molecular weight heparins (LMWH) are the agents of choice for antenatal thromboprophylaxis; dose is based on weight
- Antenatal prophylactic LMWH is offered to:
  - any woman with ≥3 risk factors listed above
  - women with previous recurrent VTE, a previous pregnancy-related VTE, or a previous VTE and family history of VTE in a first-degree relative (or documented thrombophilia)
  - Antithrombin deficiency, >1 thrombophilic defect, or additional risk factors
- Women with asymptomatic inherited or acquired thrombophilia should be monitored closely in the antenatal period

c) Postnatal Thromboprophylaxis Recommendations

- All women reassessed post-delivery for risk factors listed above
- All women encouraged to mobilize during postpartum period and avoid dehydration
- Women with ≥3 risk factors are given graduated compression stockings + LMWH
- Both warfarin and LMWH are safe when breastfeeding
- Women should be repeatedly assessed for risk factors for VTE if they develop intercurrent problems or require surgery or readmission in the postnatal period
- Consider LMWH for 1 week post-delivery in:
  - women with ≥2 risk factors listed above post-delivery
  - all women with BMI >40kg/m^2
  - all women who have had an emergency Caesarean section
  - all women post elective Caesarean section with ≥1 additional risk factors
  - all women with asymptomatic heritable or acquired thrombophilia, even if they were not receiving antenatal thromboprophylaxis (extended to 6 weeks if family history or other risk factors present)
- Consider LMWH for 6 weeks post-delivery in:
  - women with past history of VTE before the current pregnancy
  - women receiving LMWH antenatally; if they are receiving long-term anticoagulation with warfarin, this can be started when the risk of haemorrhage is low
  - women who have additional persistent risk factors, i.e. lasting more than 7 days postpartum (e.g. prolonged admission or wound infection)

Notes

....

....

....

....

....

....

....

....

....

....

....

Reference

Royal College of Obstetricians and Gynaecologists. *Reducing the Risk of Thrombosis and Embolism During Pregnancy and the Puerperium*. Green-top Guideline No.37. London: RCOSG, 2009

Chapter 3: **Cardiac and Vascular Anaesthesia**

Q1 Aortic Dissection

A 54-year-old man presents to the emergency department with intense sharp chest pain and tachycardia.

a) List differential diagnoses for this presentation (4 marks)

b) Outline appropriate imaging modalities and their positive findings if aortic dissection is suspected (9 marks)

c) How would you optimize this patient prior to transfer to a regional cardiothoracic centre? (7 marks)

Aims

Chest pain has a wide-ranging set of potential diagnoses and it is important that candidates are able to present a balanced approach to investigation of this symptom and manage the associated situations appropriately.

a) Differential Diagnoses

- Cardiac: acute MI, aortic regurgitation, myocarditis, pericarditis, aortic dissection
- Respiratory: pulmonary embolus, pneumonia, spontaneous pneumothorax, pleurisy
- Musculoskeletal: acute mechanical back pain
- Gastrointestinal: oesophageal spam or rupture, severe reflux, acute pancreatitis, obstructed or incarcerated epigastric hernia

b) Imaging Modalities

i) Chest X-ray
   - Aortic knuckle: may be obvious separation of calcified intima
   - Widened mediastinum
   - Cardiomegaly (pericardial effusion)
   - Blunting of costophrenic angle 2° to haemothorax formation

ii) Transthoracic Echocardiograph
   - Rapid and portable, and allows visualization of intimal flap in some cases
   - Provides dynamic information about cardiac function used to aid assessment of patient including presence and severity of aortic regurgitation (AR)
   - Windows may be inadequate to exclude diagnosis, especially in trauma, obesity, COPD, and severe calcific arterial disease. Results are operator dependent

iii) CT
   - Cross-sectional imaging with contrast enhancement allows diagnosis to be confirmed. 3D reconstruction allows better surgical planning for repair
   - Provides information about the extent of the dissection flap but none about the presence and severity of AR
   - Relatively quick and non-invasive, but caution in haemodynamically unstable patients

iv) MRI
   - Excellent imaging quality but slow to acquire images and therefore unsuitable for unstable patients. Avoids use of contrast
   - Can assess for presence of AR
   - Requires specialist monitoring because of magnet. Contraindicated with pacemaker or intracerebral clips

v) Aortography
  - Historical gold standard: allows good visualization of dissection flap, false lumen, and origin of branch arteries
  - Invasive and requires contrast; slow image acquisition and therefore unsuitable in unstable patients

c) Management Prior to Transfer

- ABC structured approach and IV access for fluid resuscitation
- Invasive monitoring: arterial line for beat-to-beat BP and serial ABG measurements, and central access for infusions of vasoactive substances
- Bloods (FBC, U&E, clotting, G&S, troponin)
- Collateral detailed medical history to identify suitability and patient's desire for surgery, and significant comorbidities
- Fluid resuscitation to achieve SBP adequate for organ perfusion but avoid over-resuscitation. Accepted endpoint SBP 100–110mmHg
- Analgesia
- Urinary catheter and hourly urometer bag
- BP control
  - β-blocker: first-line agent ($\downarrow$ heart rate and force of contraction). Aim is to reduce shear force around the origin of the dissection flap by avoiding tachycardia
  - Vasodilators (GTN, SNP) allow short-acting BP control to be achieved
  - Ca^{2+} channel antagonists are second-line agents

Notes

Q2 Carotid Endarterectomy

a) **Describe the course of the carotid artery (10 marks)**

b) **Compare and contrast regional and general anaesthetic techniques for carotid endarterectomy, including the advantages and disadvantages of both (10 marks)**

a) Anatomy of the Carotid Artery

- The right common carotid artery arises from the brachiocephalic artery and enters the neck deep to the omohyoid muscle
- The left common carotid artery arises directly from the aortic arch, medial to the phrenic and vagus nerves
- The arteries ascend from the thorax within the carotid sheath, between the recurrent laryngeal nerve (medial) and the vagus nerve (lateral), along with the internal jugular vein (lateral). The cervical sympathetic trunk lies just posterior and external to the sheath

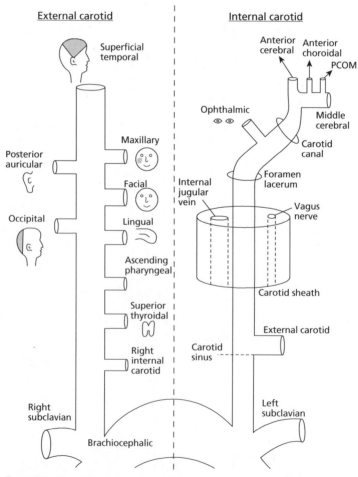

Figure 9. Carotid artery

- At the level of C4 (upper border of the thyroid cartilage) the artery divides into external and internal branches. The carotid sinus is located at this bifurcation. It contains baroreceptors (stretch receptors involved in BP regulation) and the carotid body (chemoreceptors involved in control of ventilation)

i) External Branch (ECA)
    - Supplies the upper part of the neck and the face
    - Ascends through the neck to the parotid gland and ends behind the neck of the mandible by dividing into the maxillary and superficial temporal arteries. In the neck it lies deep to the sternocleidomastoid on the lateral wall of the pharynx. Initially it lies anteromedial to the ICA and the moves to lie lateral to it with the glossopharyngeal nerve and branches of the vagus nerve between the two vessels. It has eight branches (superficial thyroid, ascending pharyngeal, lingual, facial, maxillary, occipital, posterior auricular, superficial temporal) and ends within the parotid gland:

ii) Internal Branch (ICA)
    - Supplies the orbit and provides majority of arterial supply to the brain
    - Gives off no branches within the neck
    - Initially lateral to the ECA, it moves behind the IJV to enter the middle cranial fossa via the foramen lacerum and carotid canal
    - The intracranial ICA divides into three portions:
        - petrosal: within the carotid canal in the petrous temporal bone
        - cavernous: passes through cavernous sinus, gives off branches to trigeminal ganglion
        - supraclinoid: intracranial branches (ophthalmic, posterior communicating, striate, and anterior choroidal)
    - Terminal bifurcation at the anterior perforated substance into the anterior cerebral artery and the middle cerebral artery continuing as the main body of the vessel

b) General vs. Local Anaesthetic

i) General Anaesthetic

    Advantages
    - Secure airway and control of ventilation
    - Patient preference
    - ↓ of $CMRO_2$ by induction and maintenance agents
    - Allows manipulation of temperature
    - No time constraints

    Disadvantages
    - CVS complications of induction and intubation
    - Unconscious patient requires alternative cerebral flow monitoring (labour and operator dependent)
    - ↑ use of shunts (associated with ↑ incidence of postoperative neurological dysfunction)
    - Difficulty in assessing neurological function postoperatively because of residual effects of anaesthesia and analgesia

ii) Regional Anaesthetic

    Advantages
    - Allows continual assessment of patient's neurological function and early detection of potential ischaemia
    - ↓ incidence for shunting
    - Earlier postoperative assessment possible
    - ↓ incidence of BP fluctuations and potential cardiac events

Disadvantages
- Patient cooperation required
- Surgical team must be happy to operate on an awake patient
- Patients often restless lying still for long periods (e.g. if back pain)
- Shivering if cold
- Coughing
- Need to pass urine
- Claustrophobia with drapes
- Unsecured airway
- Block complications:
  - phrenic and recurrent laryngeal nerve block
  - Horner's syndrome
  - vascular injection
  - total spinal injection
  - nerve trunk injury
  - systemic toxicity of LA
- GALA trial, published in December 2008, compared LA with GA for carotid endarterectomy. Overall no difference in primary outcomes (e.g. stroke, MI, death at <30 days)

Notes

References

Howell, S. J. (2007). Carotid endarterectomy. *British Journal of Anaesthesia*, **99**(1): 119-1–31

Lewis, S. C., C. P. Warlow CP, Bodenham AR, *et al*. (2008). General anaesthesia versus local anaesthesia for carotid surgery (GALA): a multicentre, randomised controlled trial. *Lancet Lancet*, **372**(9656): 2132-21–42

Q3 Cervical Plexus

a) **Describe the cervical plexus (9 marks)**

b) **What regional anaesthetic techniques would you employ for awake carotid endarterectomy surgery? (11 marks)**

Aims

A less commonly encountered piece of anatomy in the final examination, the cervical plexus is relatively straightforward to reproduce and has obvious clinical indications. Also, only a few techniques are used to block it, unlike other nerve plexuses commonly encountered in the examination, and it is well worth practising this question despite the recent GALA trial showing no obvious benefit to carotid surgery performed under regional technique.

a) Cervical Plexus

- Unification of the upper four cervical anterior nerve roots (sensory) and upper five cervical anterior nerve roots (motor)
- Broadly divided into motor and sensory

  Motor

  Four main branches exist
  - Ansa cervicalis: roots C1–3
    - Superior root (C1): geniohyoid and thyrohyoid
    - Inferior root (C2, 3): omohyoid, sternothyroid, and sternohyoid
  - Branch to longus capitis and collis: C2-4
  - Phrenic nerve: C3–5 motor to diaphragm
  - Accessory cranial nerve: C2–5 motor to sternocleidomastoid and trapezius

  Sensory

  Four main branches exist
  - Greater auricular nerve
  - Transverse cervical nerve
  - Lesser occipital nerve
  - Supraclavicular nerve

  Root values for all: C2–4

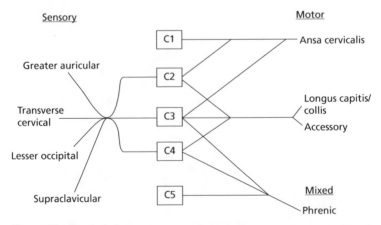

Figure 10. Cervical plexus

b) Regional Anaesthesia

- Requires blockade of the superficial and deep cervical plexi
- LA supplementation by the surgeon is usually required, especially at carotid sheath
- In addition, a submental block may be performed

Superficial Plexus Block

- Infiltration along the posterior border of sternocleidomastoid muscle to block lesser occipital nerve, greater auricular nerve, anterior cutaneous nerve, and supraclavicular nerve

Deep Cervical Plexus Block

- Patient turns head away from side of block with neck extended
- Palpate C6 transverse process (Chaissaignac's tubercle) at level of cricoid cartilage
- Locate the same point at C2 (inferior to mastoid process) and draw a line
- The transverse processes of C3 and C4 lie at equal points along this line
- A needle is directed caudally and medially until the relevant transverse process is encountered, withdrawn slightly, and aspirated.
- A test dose of 1mL of LA is injected to ensure correct placement and then the remaining volume is injected
- Two techniques exist
  - Multiple-shot techniques: C2, C3, and C4 transverse processes are identified with three separate needles and 5mL of LA injected at each level
  - Single shot technique: C4 transverse process located as above and 10–15mL of LA is injected at this level
- Recent descriptions of ultrasound-guided techniques have shown that they require lower rates of surgical supplementation
- Nerve stimulator can be incorporated looking for stimulation of the occipital muscles as an appropriate response

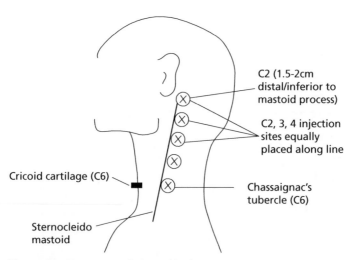

Figure 11. Deep cervical plexus block

Notes

Q4 Cardiopulmonary Bypass 1

a) What is a cardiopulmonary bypass (CPB) circuit? (6 marks)

b) Describe the different components and functions of a standard cardiopulmonary bypass circuit (14 marks)

Aims

Although not contributing hugely to the SAQ section recently, cardiac topics such as this may just as easily crop up in the SOE section. Candidates should have an understanding of the CPB circuit because of the potential physiological changes that it can inflict on the patient

a) Definition

- The machinery that replicates the function of the heart and lungs, allowing the native cardiorespiratory function to be stopped, thus creating a bloodless and motionless field for surgery
- Most CPB circuits drain under gravity via large-bore catheters from the venous circulation (e.g. right atrium or SVC)
- Return line via arterial cannula to systemic circulation (e.g. thoracic aorta)
- The circuit is coated with a variety of compounds to reduce activation of coagulation and inflammatory cascades
  - Heparin: inhibits thrombogenic response of blood to the circuit, and ↓ clot formation (↓ total heparin dose required), ↓ A–a gradient, and ↓ pulmonary vascular resistance
  - Phosphorylcholine: anti-inflammatory and antithrombotic properties; aims to replicate cell membrane surface on circuit

b) CPB Circuit

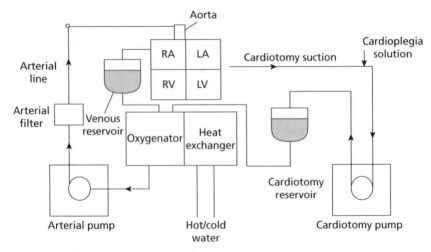

Figure 12. Cardiopulmonary bypass circuit

i) Reservoirs
- Venous: receives blood under gravity from a venous cannula and surgical suction
- Cardiotomy: receives blood from a low-volume displacement cannula placed in the left ventricle to prevent accumulation of blood, chamber distension, and subendocardial ischaemia

ii) Oxygenator
- Most modern circuits use membrane oxygenators
- Fresh gas flows through the middle of multiple fine capillary tubes around which blood circulates
- The FiO_2 determines the partial pressure of O_2; fresh gas flow acts as a sweep gas to determine the $PaCO_2$. Fresh gas flow is inversely related to the $PaCO_2$
- Efficency falls with use: microthrombi and proteinaceous debris decrease the surface area available for gas exchange
- Heparin-coated oxygenators are associated with ↑ postoperative platelet counts

iii) Heat exchanger
- Allows manipulation of blood temperature from reservoirs to alter core temperature of patient
- Allows therapeutic hypothermia during bypass and resuscitation of refractory hypothermia

iv) Pumps
- Suction blood from the venous and cardiotomy reservoirs, and direct it into the oxygenator and heat exchanger
- Centrifugal devices commonly used (previously used roller pumps but thought to trigger cell damage and inflammation)

v) Arterial filter
- Removes gaseous and particulate emboli from blood: ↓ microvascular occlusion and complications from CPB, pore size 27–40µm
- Specialized leucocyte depletion filters shown to produce slight ↓ in renal injury post-bypass

Notes

References

De Somer F. Impact of oxygenator characteristics on its capability to remove gaseous microemboli. *Journal of Extra-Corporeal Technology*, **39**: 271–3, 2007

Jameel S, Colah S, Klein AA. Recent advances in cardiopulmonary bypass techniques. *Continuing Education in Anaesthesia, Critical Care & Pain*, **10**: 20–3, 2010

Sohn N, Marcoux J, Mycyk T, Krahn J, Meng Q. The impact of different biocompatible coated cardiopulmonary bypass circuits on inflammatory response and oxidative stress. *Perfusion*, **24**: 231–7, 2009

Q5 Cardiopulmonary Bypass 2

a) List the clinical indications for cardiopulmonary bypass (CPB) (5 marks)

b) Outline the complications associated with CPB (15 marks)

Aims

The complications following CPB are well documented and are a popular topic in both the written and oral sections of the examination. In addition, they feature regularly in postoperative bypass patients and a level of detail will be required even if you have not managed this cohort extensively.

a) Indications for CPB

i) Theatre
  - Heart valve surgery
  - On-pump coronary artery bypass grafting
  - Structural heart surgery (e.g. correction of congenital defects)
  - Pulmonary vasculature surgery
  - Proximal thoracic aorta surgery
  - Deep induced hypothermia (commonly 22–28°C, although some clinicians use 15°C)

ii) ICU
  - For respiratory failure (venovenous extra-corporeal membrane oxygenation)
  - For cardiovascular failure (arteriovenous extra-corporeal membrane oxygenation)
  - Rewarming of refractory hypothermia
  - Refractory cardiogenic shock
  - As a bridge to transplant in endstage cardiac failure

b) Complications Associated with CPB

i) Circuit-related
  - Platelet activation
  - Activation of clotting cascades and complement pathways
  - Cell damage
  - Particulate or gas emboli formation
  - Cannulation:
    - Venous:
      - haemorrhage
      - organ or vessel damage
      - ↓ preload
      - air embolism during cannula insertion
    - Aortic:
      - haemorrhage
      - emboli of atherosclerotic plaque or air into arterial circulation
      - dissection
      - malpositioning of cannula

ii) Patient-related
  - Overall incidence 0.5–1%: often transient and subtle

Central nervous system
- Focal neurological abnormalities (1–6% patients postoperatively)
  - Main form of neurological complications from CPB
  - Hemiparesis, sensory neural hearing loss, or visual field defects
  - Risk factors: ↑ age, premorbid cerebrovascular or carotid artery disease, valve surgery, poor preoperative LV function, long bypass times
- Global neurological abnormality (3% cases)
  - Overall ↓ level of awareness 1–3 days postoperatively
  - Non-sedative persistent coma >24 hours postoperatively is a significant mortality risk factor
  - Neuropsychological, i.e. early postoperative emotional, memory, and attention defects

Respiratory
- Atelectasis is commonplace, especially if the pleura is opened for internal mammary grafting
- ↑ A–a gradient and ↓ FRC:
  - Shunt, hypoxaemia, and ↑ requirement for ventilation
  - ALI or ARDS may be seen in 1–2% of cases
- Sputum retention common post-sternotomy: ↑ risk for pneumonia, especially if comorbid respiratory disease exists

Cardiovascular system
- Post-bypass cardiac function relates to preoperative state
- Ventricle is often stiff with ↓ lusitropy immediately postoperatively; tolerates bradycardia poorly
- Arrhythmias are common (hypoxia or electrolyte abnormalities); pacing wires are routinely placed to treat bradyarrhythmias
- Low vascular tone is common immediately postoperatively, requiring vasopressors to maintain MAP

Gastrointestinal (<2%)
- 20% of patients have postoperative elevated bilirubin
- Risk of upper GI bleed is higher; postoperative peak around 10 days
- Pancreatitis may be triggered by hypothermia
- Risk of ischaemic bowel due to emboli showering into the GI arterial tree

Renal
- 1–4% of patients; often reversible
- Significant predictor of mortality, especially if requiring renal support therapy
- ↑ risk: pre-existing renal disease, ↑ age, long bypass times, poor cardiac output

Other
- Poor platelet function and coagulopathy: require transfusion of PRC and clotting products
- Peripheral insulin resistance is commonplace with poor glucose control
- ↑ in total body water due to increased capillary permeability is often seen
- Embolic occlusion and compartment syndrome are theoretical but rare complications
- General myopathy, especially in patients who remain in the ICU and are ventilated

Notes

....

....

....

....

....

....

....

....

....

....

....

Reference

Jameel S, Colah S, Klein AA. Recent advances in cardiopulmonary bypass techniques. *Continuing Education in Anaesthesia, Critical Care & Pain*, **10**: 20–3, 2010

Q6 Dilated Cardiomyopathy

You have been asked to anaesthetise a 68-year-old man for a right inguinal hernia repair. He is also under the care of the cardiologists for a dilated cardiomyopathy

a) List the causes of a dilated cardiomyopathy (5 marks)

b) What signs and symptoms are characteristic of this disease? (5 marks)

c) Outline important factors to consider when anaesthetising this patient (10 marks)

Aims

As medicine advances patients are being considered for surgery despite significant medical comorbidities, and an understanding of how to assess and investigate these cohorts is being examined in this question. Guidelines for assessment of these groups have been published by many colleges, and these are an excellent way of structuring if available.

a) Causes

- Cardiac ischaemia
- Cardiac valvular abnormalities
- Post-viral infection
- Associated with other comorbidities (e.g. chronic alcoholism, sickle cell disease, muscular dystrophy, hypothyroidism, drugs (i.e. chemotherapy))
- Idiopathic

b) Signs and Symptoms

- Tachycardia (low cardiac output state)
- Arrhythmias
- Cardiac failure (e.g. peripheral oedema, dyspnoea, ascites)
- Mitral and/or tricuspid regurgitation
- Embolus formation (intracardiac more likely)
- Worsening systolic or diastolic function and ↑ LVEDP on echocardiography

c) Anaesthesia

i) Preoperative
- Liaise with the cardiologists to ensure optimal medical treatment (e.g. ACE inhibitors, angiotensin II inhibitors, diuretics, β-blockers, anticoagulation if emboli risk high)
- Consider biventricular pacing if poor response to pharmacological therapies
- Preoperative investigations: ECG to look at ischaemia and arrhythmias, and echocardiography to look at valves, systolic and diastolic function, and ejection fraction
- Aggressive treatment or correction of arrhythmias (e.g. AF and electrolyte abnormalities)

ii) Intraoperative
- Establish invasive arterial blood pressure monitoring prior to induction of anaesthesia. Have a low threshold for CVP monitoring
- Consider regional anaesthesia, especially good for this hernia case (care with under-perfusion of coronary vessels secondary to hypotension)

- Maximize coronary perfusion by avoiding tachycardia, judicious use of drugs with a negative inotropic effect (e.g. induction agents), and careful use of inotropes or vasopressors
- Prevent sympathetic surges and increased afterload with adequate depth of anaesthesia, muscle relaxation if appropriate, and good analgesia
- In patients with raised LVEDP, maintain adequate preload with IV fluid administration

iii) Postoperative
- If straightforward operation under purely regional technique, could return to ward after prolonged monitoring in recovery
- Otherwise, HDU or ICU to maximize BP, HR, rhythm control, optimal fluid management, tissue oxygenation, and analgesia (consider further regional techniques for prolonged effect)

Notes

....

....

....

....

....

....

....

....

....

....

....

Reference

Davies MR, Cousins J. Cardiomyopathy and anaesthesia. *Continuing Education in Anaesthesia, Critical Care & Pain*, **9**: 189–93, 2009

Q7 EndoVascular Aneurysm Repair (EVAR)

a) Discuss different techniques for anaesthetising an endovascular aneurysm repair (EVAR) for an abdominal aortic aneurysm, including the advantages and disadvantages of each (10 marks)

b) Outline significant complications associated with the EVAR approach (10 marks)

Aims

Abdominal aortic aneurysm (AAA) can now be definitively treated by means of endovascular stenting. Candidates should be familiar with management of EVAR and the issues pertinent to anaesthetising these high-risk patients in a remote site.

a) Anaesthetic Techniques

- Invasive arterial monitoring (usually right radial cannulation as radiological access to the left axillary artery is sometimes required), large-bore IV access, urinary catheter. CVP line insertion not routinely required
- Surgery is usually performed in a combined radiology–surgery suite, often separate from theatres with delayed levels of anaesthetic support
- Bilateral longitudinal incisions expose the femoral arteries for stent deployment
- Research shows potential advantages in RA techniques over GA: a reduction in ICU bed usage and hospital length of stay, and a lower incidence of postoperative morbidity (e.g. renal failure) and mortality

i) Local anaesthesia
- Adequate topical analgesia can be achieved using local infiltration
- Greater risk of poor patient compliance
- Avoids complications of GA
- Some studies show a lower incidence of renal failure

ii) Regional Anaesthesia (± sedation, e.g. TCI propofol)
- Subarachnoid (both single-shot and continuous), combined spinal–epidural (CSE), or epidural anaesthesia. The latter two techniques allow the block to be topped up during long cases and can be used for postoperative analgesia
- Perioperative anticoagulation is required during these cases, which poses a theoretical risk of central neuraxial haematoma formation
- Compliance is important: during screening for the presence of a type I endoleak (failure of the stent graft to seal at the proximal and distal landing zones), the patient must remain still and hold their breath
- May be a challenge to maintain compliance for extended cases (>3 hours)

iii) General Anaesthetic
- Significant cardiorespiratory comorbidity in this cohort makes RA preferable; thorough preoperative assessment for suitability for GA is required
- Avoids patients being awake and stressed by procedure
- No constraints on surgical time
- Requires additional postoperative analgesia to be addressed

b) Complications

i) Immediate
- Aneurysm rupture
- Conversion to open (quoted as 2%)

- Endoleak: defined as failure to isolate the aneurysm sac with the graft (5–10%)
- Vessel dissection
- Poor distal flow and ischaemia
- Distal emboli
- Neurological insult (anterior spinal artery occlusion, spinal cord infarction)

ii) Early
- Peri- and postoperative arrhythmias, myocardial ischaemia, and cardiac failure
- Peri- and postoperative respiratory complications (lobar collapse, hypoxia, and pneumonia)
- Peri- and postoperative renal failure
- Endoleak
- Graft occlusion or displacement
- Post-implantation syndrome; characterized by fever and elevated CRP and WCC in the absence of infection. Usually lasts 2–10 days and responds to NSAIDs

iii) Delayed
- Stent displacement
- Stent fracture
- Venous thromboembolism
- Recurrence of aneurysm

The EndoVascular Aneurysm Repair (EVAR) trials were instigated to assess the safety and efficacy of endovascular aneurysm repair in the treatment of AAA in terms of mortality, quality of life, durability, and cost-effectiveness for patients considered fit for open repair (EVAR Trial 1) or unfit for open repair (EVAR Trial 2). Following their results, NICE Guidelines were updated in 2009 to suggest that EVAR is reserved for elective patients and is not used in the treatment of ruptured aneurysms

Notes

....

....

....

....

....

....

References

Pichel AC, Serracino-Inglott F. Anaesthetic considerations for endovascular abdominal aortic aneurysm repair (EVAR). *Current Anaesthesia & Critical Care*, **19**: 150–162, 2008

Sadat, U., Cooper DG, Gillard JH, Walsh SR, Hayes PD. Impact of the type of anesthesia on outcome after elective endovascular aortic aneurysm repair: literature review. *Vascular*, **16**: 340–5, 2008

http://www.evartrials.org/index.htm (accessed 15 June 2010)

http://www.nice.org.uk/nicemedia/pdf/TA167QRG.pdf (accessed 15 June 2010)

Q8 Intra-Aortic Balloon Pump

a) List the indications and contraindications for inserting an intra-aortic balloon pump (IABP) (7 marks)

b) Describe the mechanism of action and physiological effects of an IABP (6 marks)

c) What are the potential complications of IABP insertion? (7 marks)

Aims

Candidates may have to look after patients with an IABP and therefore must understand the physiology behind their actions. The topic may extend to the physical principles encountered when using this device.

a) Indications

- Unstable angina
- Acute myocardial ischaemia or infarction
- Acute mechanical complication of MI (e.g. mitral regurgitation)
- Ventricular septal defect
- Ventricular arrhythmias
- Cardiogenic shock
- Refractory ventricular failure
- Weaning from cardiopulmonary bypass
- As a bridge to cardiac transplant
- High-risk percutaneous transluminal coronary angioplasty
- Complicated paediatric congenital cardiac abnormalities

b) Contraindications

i) Absolute
- Patient refusal
- Irreversible or endstage cardiac disease
- Moderate to severe aortic regurgitation
- Aortic dissection
- Presence of aortic stents

ii) Relative
- Severe neurological deficit
- Compromising tachyarrhythmias
- Abdominal aortic aneurysm
- Severe peripheral vascular disease

b) IABP

- The IABP, pioneered at the Grace-Sinai Hospital in Detroit in the early 1960s, is a device used to augment failing hearts
- An intra-arterial device is placed in the thoracic aorta, usually via the femoral artery, distal to the left subclavian artery and proximal to the renal arteries
- The device consists of a catheter with a balloon and pressure transducer
- During diastole, the balloon is inflated with helium, isolating a column of blood between the aortic valve and the tip of the balloon
- Subsequent elastic recoil in the aortic wall results in ↑ pressure which is transmitted to the coronary artery origins, increasing the diastolic perfusion gradient

i) Primary effects
- Increased coronary perfusion and subsequent oxygen delivery
- Reduced myocardial oxygen demand

ii) Secondary effects
- ↓ SVR immediately following deflation of the balloon, promoting forward flow, resulting in ↑ ejection fraction, reducing end-diastolic volume and wall tension
- These two factors combined can result in ↑ cardiac output, ↓ heart rate, and ↓ myocardial lactate production

c) Complications

- Damage to vessels
  - ◆ False aneurysm
  - ◆ Aortic dissection
  - ◆ Haematoma formation
  - ◆ Vessels supplying the GI tract, with subsequent gut ischaemia
- Damage to adjacent structures
  - ◆ Limb ischaemia
  - ◆ Limb compartment syndrome
  - ◆ Loss of peripheral pulses
  - ◆ Cardiac tamponade
- Balloon effects
  - ◆ Rupture: helium embolus formation
  - ◆ Immobility: balloons become lodged in position
  - ◆ Malposition: cerebral or renal circulation problems
- Other
  - ◆ Local, e.g. infection, bleeding, thrombus formation
  - ◆ Emboli formation

Notes

Reference

Krishna M, Zacharowski K. Principles of intra-aortic balloon pump counterpulsation. *Continuing Education in Anaesthesia, Critical Care & Pain.* **9**: 24–8, 2009

Q9 **Long QT Syndrome**

You are asked to anaesthetise a 34-year-old woman with long QT syndrome for a knee arthroscopy.

a) **List the causes of long QT syndrome (6 marks)**

b) **What cardiovascular risks exist with long QT syndrome? (2 marks)**

c) **Outline relevant factors for consideration when anaesthetising this patient (12 marks)**

Aims

Although long QT syndrome is quite rare, candidates should be aware of the potential problems that technique and choice of drugs may have on patients with this syndrome.

a) Causes

i) Congenital
  * Jervell-Lange-Nielsen syndrome: autosomal recessive, associated with varying cardiac symptoms, congenital deafness, and sudden death
  * Romano–Ward syndrome: autosomal dominant

ii) Acquired
  * Electrolyte imbalance
  * Severe nutritional deficit (e.g. anorexia)
  * Sympathetic stimulation (e.g. pain, subarachnoid haemorrhage)
  * Hypothermia
  * Drugs which cause torsades de pointes:
    ◆ antiarrhythmics (e.g. sotalol, flecainide, amiodarone, quinidine, procainamide)
    ◆ antimicrobials and antifungals (e.g. erythromycin, clarithromycin, fluconazole)
    ◆ antipsychotics/antidepressants (e.g. chlorpromazine, fluoxetine, haloperidol)

b) Cardiovascular Risks

* Mutations of cardiac ion channels causing inadequate ventricular repolarization
* Risk of developing malignant ventricular arrhythmias (e.g. torsades de pointes)
* Arrhythmias spontaneously return to sinus rhythm or progress into potentially fatal VF

c) Anaesthetic Considerations

* Aim is to avoid precipitation of potentially harmful ventricular arrhythmias

i) Preoperative
  * Anaesthetic history and examination, including previous CVS symptoms, attacks, and treatment
  * Preoperative ECG to assess QT and QT_c interval (may be normal in some patients)
  * Cardiology review and optimization of medication: continuation of β-blocker medication perioperatively (adequate if Valsalva manoeuvre does not alter QT_c interval)
  * Preoperative U&Es with correction if required

ii) Intraoperative
  * Aim is to minimize development of arrhythmias by limiting the surgical stress response
    ◆ Consider sedative premedication
    ◆ Obtund the pressor response to airway instrumentation using opioids (e.g. alfentanil)

     ◆ Adequate analgesia: consider a regional technique here
     ◆ IPPV to minimize hypercapnia and ↑ intrathoracic pressures
- Avoidance of hypothermia with active warming devices
- Consider invasive blood pressure measurement for electrolyte monitoring
- Avoid drugs which prolong the QT_c interval and may precipitate arrhythmias (e.g. ketamine, suxamethonium, atropine, glycopyrrolate, neostigmine)
- Have necessary resuscitation and pacing equipment available
- Treat arrhythmias promptly: if torsades de pointes develops, IV magnesium sulphate 2g over 20min, repeat, and then commence an infusion of 3–20mg/min if no improvement

iii) Postoperative
- Continuous ECG monitoring until awake (or for longer if larger procedure)
- Adequate analgesia
- Ask for as calm an environment as possible!

Notes

Reference

Hunter JD, Sharma P, Rathi S. Long QT syndrome. *Continuing Education in Anaesthesia, Critical Care & Pain*, **8**: 67–70, 2008

Q10 Pacemaker Indications

a) List the indications for insertion of a pacemaker (6 marks)

b) Define the nomenclature system used in modern pacemaker devices (7 marks)

c) List the potential complications associated with a patient undergoing non-cardiac surgery with a permanent pacemaker *in situ* (7 marks)

Aims

Patients with pacemakers frequently present for all forms of surgery. Candidates must be able to decipher the type of pacemaker and what effect this has on anaesthesia, whilst understanding the wider issues of comorbid cardiac disease and the safety issues these devices present.

a) Pacemaker Insertion

i) Temporary
   - Associated with an acute MI:
     - asystole
     - second- or third-degree heart block with symptoms or following an anterior MI
     - new trifasicular block
   - Not associated with an acute MI:
     - symptomatic junctional bradycardia
     - tachycardic or bradycardic syndrome with symptomatic pauses
   - Prophylactic:
     - preoperative patients with second- or third-degree heart block, bi- or trifascicular block
   - Following cardiac surgery
   - Following failure of a permanent system

ii) Permanent
   - Symptomatic second- or third-degree heart block
   - Tachycardic or bradycardic syndrome with symptomatic pauses
   - Post cardiac transplant with bradyarrythmias
   - Paroxysmal supraventricular tachyarrhythmias

b) Pacemaker Nomenclature

Chamber paced	Chamber sensed	Response	Rate response	Anti-tachycardia function
O – none	O – none	O – none	O – none	O – none
A – Atrium	A – Atrium	I – Inhibit	R – Adapt	P – ATP
V – Ventricle	V – Ventricle	T – Trigger		S – Shock
D – Dual	D – Dual	D – Dual		D – Dual
S – Single	S – Single			

c) Perioperative Complications

i) Preoperative
   - Indication for pacemaker: may represent significant cardiac disease
   - Ask the patient to see their pacemaker card to confirm timing of last pacemaker check and modification of functions for surgery (e.g. defibrillation function)
   - Have a low threshold for arranging a pacemaker check if not done recently

ii) Intraoperative
- Suxamethonium: fasiculations may be interpreted either as VF and trigger inappropriate shock delivery, or as representing electrical activity with subsequent discharge
- Diathermy: may be detected by pacemaker as native cardiac activity, inhibiting or activating functions
  - If constant interference isdetected, the pacemaker should default to VVI
  - Risk of micro-shock along the pacing leads
  - Can char the pacing wire insertion points, thereby ↑ the threshold and ↓ capture peri- and postoperatively
- Use of a magnet in modern pacemakers has less predictable responses
- Defibrillation pads should not be placed directly over the pacemaker (>12cm from the generator is the currently recommended minimum safe distance)
- Avoid use of N_2O in a recently implanted pacemaker as accumulation can cause detachment of the anode lead in unipolar pacemakers

iii) Postoperative
- Pacemaker check ± reactivation of the programmable functions may be warranted
- Shivering can cause myopotential generation which may be interpreted as cardiac activity

Notes

Q11 Ruptured Abdominal Aortic Aneurysm

You are called by the surgeons to see a 78-year-old man in the Emergency Department with abdominal pain. CT abdomen demonstrates a leaking abdominal aortic aneurysm (AAA). His BP is 90/45mmHg. There is no vascular surgeon on call in your hospital.

a) Who should be involved in making the decision on whether to operate on this patient? (6 marks)

b) List the preoperative factors associated with good and bad outcomes (8 marks)

c) Assuming that the decision to operate has been made, discuss the preparation of this patient for transfer to a hospital with vascular cover (6 marks)

Aims

Whilst the management of a ruptured AAA has featured in recent SAQ papers, we felt it important to cover other aspects of this type of case. Emphasis is on discussion between senior clinicians from multidisciplinary backgrounds.

a) Decision to Operate

This is a multidisciplinary decision, involving the patient if appropriate
- Consultant anaesthetist
- Consultant general surgeon
- Regional vascular surgeon on call
- Patient, if deemed mentally competent; if not, discuss with next of kin, but they are unable to consent. A lack of competence may indicate poor prognosis

b) Perioperative Factors

i) Good Outcome
- Preoperative serum creatinine <130mmol/L
- Evidence of good preoperative urine output
- Presence of an infra-renal aneurysm, compared with supra- or juxta-renal
- Lack of cardiorespiratory comorbidities

ii) Bad Outcome
- Preoperative comorbidities (e.g. chronic renal failure, ischaemic heart disease, COPD)
- Intraperitoneal rupture
- Persistent preoperative hypotension, i.e. systolic BP <90mmHg
- Evidence of multi-organ complications
- Hardman study: a retrospective study which identified five variables associated with poor outcome:
  - age >76 years
  - ischaemic ECG
  - creatinine >190mmol/L
  - low GCS
  - Hb <9g/dL
- If >3 variables were present, associated with 100% mortality

c) Transfer Preparation

- Transfer may not worsen outcome and some patients remain stable for a period of time post-leaking
- Clinical issues: aim to keep systolic BP between 90 and 95mmHg with judicious fluid administration; avoid hypertension and the risk of complete aneurysmal rupture
- Invasive arterial monitoring and wide-bore venous access is mandatory for transfer
- Have pre-drawn up vasoactive drugs available prior to transfer
- Investigations: FBC, U&E, clotting, cross-matched blood to be available for transfer
- Copies of all blood tests, ECGs, X-rays, and CT scans
- Appropriate accompanying medical personnel to be discussed; many district general hospitals do not send an anaesthetist with the patient as standard
- Consider whether the patient is appropriate for radiological intervention with endovascular grafting

Notes

References

Adam DJ, Mohan IV, Stuart WP, Bain M, Bradbury AW. Community and hospital outcome from ruptured abdominal aortic aneurysm within the catchment area of a regional vascular surgical service. *Journal of Vascular Surgery*, **30**: 922–8, 1999

Hardman DT, Fisher CM, Patel MI, *et al.* Ruptured abdominal aortic aneurysms: who should be offered surgery? *Journal of Vascular Surgery*, **23**: 123–9, 1996

Q12 Tamponade

You are asked to review a 63-year-old man who has become hypotensive 5 hours post-CABG. You are concerned that the patient is developing cardiac tamponade.

a) List further clinical features to support your diagnosis (5 marks)

b) What investigations will confirm a diagnosis of cardiac tamponade? (4 marks)

c) Describe your immediate management of this patient (11 marks)

Aims

This is a true cardiothoracic emergency, and requires vigilance and teamwork with cardiothoracic surgeons to prevent further clinical deterioration. With this in mind, a well-structured answer to this question is required to convince the examiners of your ability to diagnose and manage this scenario.

a) Clinical Features

- Classically: Beck's triad of hypotension, raised JVP, and 'muffled' heart sounds
- Hypotension resistant to fluids and inotropes
- Pulsus paradoxus (absent if severe LV dysfunction), Kussmaul's sign (rise in JVP during inspiration), pericardial friction rub
- Pleuritic chest pain, dyspnoea
- Oliguria and metabolic acidosis may also be present
- If pulmonary artery catheter *in situ*, equalization of pressures of atria and LVEDP

b) Investigations

- Gold standard: transoesophageal echocardiography (if patient sedated and ventilated)
  - Presence of 1cm of pericardial separation in an unexplained clinical deterioration is sensitive in detecting tamponade
  - Transthoracic echocardiography is more unreliable
- CXR: widened mediastinum and globular cardiac silhouette, but difficult to interpret
- ECG: may show pulsus alternans or small-voltage QRS complexes

c) Management

- In this patient, tamponade is due to excess mediastinal bleeding and accumulation of pericardiac clot, leading to cardiac chamber compression and cardiac output reduction
- Only option is re-sternotomy under GA to drain the pericardium and remove the clot. Requires a senior anaesthetist, preferably with cardiothoracic experience
- Needle pericardiocentesis will not remove all clot and risks damaging grafted vessels
- If patient is stable enough, transfer to theatre for optimal conditions; very occasionally the patient may require sternotomy on the ICU if too unstable to move
- Ensure cross-matched blood is available prior to transfer
- If awake, give 15L/min O_2 by non-rebreather face mask; if sedated, ensure adequate oxygenation, ventilation, and sedation for transfer to theatre
- Transfer to theatre with full invasive monitoring, fluids, and inotropes as required
- If already ventilated, transfer to theatre ventilator and maintain anaesthesia with volatile or IV agent of choice and administer muscle relaxation
- An awake patient represents a significant challenge because of the sudden loss of sympathetic drive maintaining cardiac output on induction of anaesthesia

- Induce anaesthesia on the operating table with the patient 'prepped' and draped:
  - IV opiate (e.g. fentanyl 2–10mcg/kg)
  - Induction agent (e.g. thiopental 1–4mg/kg or etomidate 0.1–0.2 mg/kg)
  - Neuromuscular blocker (e.g. suxamethonium 1–2mg/kg, rocuronium 0.6–1mg/kg)
- Obtain a baseline ABG and thromboelastography sample
- NB: Upon sternal opening and drainage of pericardial tamponade, inotrope requirements may fall considerably because of improved cardiac pumping efficiency and output, and endogenous catecholamine release

Notes

Chapter 4: **Neuroanaesthesia and Neurointensive Care**

Q1 Circle of Willis

a) **Describe the anatomy of the circle of Willis (7 marks)**

b) **List the different causes of cerebral aneurysms and outline the most common locations for these aneurysms within this circulation (6 marks)**

c) **What signs and symptoms may be described in the history and examination of a patient with a suspected subarachnoid haemorrhage (SAH)? (7 marks)**

Aims

This should be an area of anatomy that you can confidently reproduce, possibly with the aid of a diagram similar to the one shown. The obvious questions usually associated with the anatomy are well covered in previous texts. Therefore we have linked this to the extensive topic of subarachnoid haemorrhage.

a) Circle of Willis

- The anastomosis of blood vessels found at the base of the brain that are responsible for arterial flow to the brain and brainstem
- Formed by the unification of the anterior and posterior circulations
- The anterior circulation is formed from the internal carotid artery, which gives off five branches within the cranial cavity
- The posterior communicating artery joins with the posterior cerebral artery to form the other half of the circle
- The anterior communicating artery completes this ring, branching from the two anterior cerebral arteries

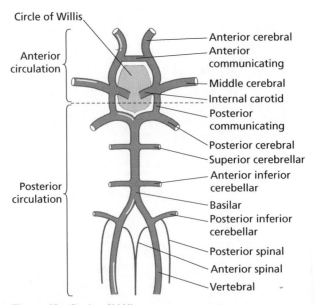

Figure 13. Circle of Willis

b) Aneurysms

- An aneurysm is an abnormal local dilatation in the wall of a blood vessel, usually an artery, due to a defect, disease, or injury
  - ◆ Saccular: the most common, resulting from local medial degeneration following haemodynamic-induced vascular injury. Mainly occurs at bifurcation of large vessels
  - ◆ Fusiform: found in older patients. Caused by unusual and excessive atherosclerotic breakdown on the intima
  - ◆ Dissecting: results in accumulation of blood within the wall of the vessel between the intima and elastic lamina. Arises either spontaneously or following trauma. Also found in patients with underlying vasculopathies, usually within the vertebral artery
  - ◆ Other: arteriovenous malformations, vasculitides, tumours
- Nearly 90% of aneurysms are found in the anterior circulation (carotid), anterior and posterior communicating arteries, and middle cerebral arteries
- Less than 20% are found in the posterior circulation (vertebrobasilar)

c) SAH Signs and Symptoms

- Sudden-onset headache: 'worst-ever', 'like being hit on back of head'
- Seizures
- Focal neurological signs (e.g. cranial nerve palsies)
- Fluctuating, reduction in, or loss of consciousness
- Meningism
- Nausea and vomiting
- Hunt and Hess scale
  Measures clinical severity of haemorrhage on admission (correlates well with outcome)
  - Grade 0: unruptured aneurysm
  - Grade 1: asymptomatic or minimal headache and slight nuchal rigidity
  - Grade 2: moderate to severe headache, nuchal rigidity, no neurological deficit other than cranial nerve palsy
  - Grade 3: drowsiness, confusion, or mild focal deficit
  - Grade 4: stupor, moderate to severe hemiparesis, possible early decerebrate rigidity, and vegetative disturbances
  - Grade 5: deep coma, decerebrate rigidity, and moribund appearance

Notes

Reference

Priebe HJ Aneurysmal subarachnoid haemorrhage and the anaesthetist. *British Journal of Anaesthesia*, **99**: 102–18, 2007

Q2 Head Injury

You have been called to the Emergency Department to assess a patient with an isolated head injury following an assault.

a) List the criteria for intubation and ventilation in a patient with a head injury (9 marks)

b) Describe the preparation required for safe transfer of a patient with a head injury to a tertiary neurosurgical unit (11 marks)

Aims

There are many interventions that anaesthetists can provide to prevent or minimize secondary brain injury in such patients. It is vital that candidates can recognize at what point further support is required and manage patients for transfer to tertiary centres.

a) Intubation and Ventilation

- Ensure that the cervical spine remains immobilized during manual ventilation and airway instrumentation
- Immediately if:
  - GCS ≤8
  - loss of protective laryngeal reflexes or high risk of aspiration
  - evidence of ventilatory insufficiency despite high-flow oxygen therapy (PaO_2 <13kPa, $PaCO_2$ >6kPa)
  - spontaneous hyperventilation with $PaCO_2$ <4kPa
  - irregular respirations
- Intubate prior to transfer if:
  - significantly deteriorating conscious level (even if GCS >8)
  - evidence of unstable facial fractures
  - excessive bleeding into the mouth
  - seizures

b) Transfer Preparation

- Ensure clear and detailed ongoing communication with neurosurgeon and neurosurgery centre
- Although thorough assessment and resuscitation is paramount, the priority is often a rapid transfer for neurosurgical intervention

i) Airway
- As above

ii) Breathing
- Ensure adequate sedation, analgesia, and muscle relaxation
- Aim for PaO_2 >13kPa and $PaCO_2$ 4.5–5.0kPa
- Hyperventilate with ↑FiO_2 if radiological or clinical evidence of ↑ICP
- Ensure inspired gases are humidified using a disposable heat–moisture exchange (HME) filter

iii) Cardiovascular
- Obtain wide-bore venous access and take blood samples including cross-match
- Insert an arterial cannula for invasive BP monitoring and ABG sampling

- Maintain MAP ≥80mmHg with fluids ± vasopressors if required
- If time, obtain central venous access, ideally the subclavian or femoral approach
- Catheterize the patient's bladder (urinary retention may lead to ↑ ICP)

iv) Disability
- Avoid obstruction of cerebral venous drainage, i.e. patient is nursed and transferred in a 30° reverse-Trendelenburg position, secure the endotracheal tube with tape
- Regular reassessment of pupillary reaction and size

v) Everything Else
- Insert a nasogastric or orogastric tube and allow free drainage
- Check blood glucose levels: may require insulin infusion if grossly deranged (persistent hyperglycaemia is associated with secondary brain injury and a poor outcome)
- Ensure that there is a trained and experienced assistant for the ambulance transfer
- Check that the transfer bag is fully stocked, including a mobile phone for communication, spare batteries, infusion pumps, spare money, etc.
- Enclose hard or DVD/CD copies of all radiological investigations for tertiary centre
- Ensure clear notes are maintained at all times, including standard transport documentation
- Communication with neurosurgical unit regarding time of leaving and up-to-date clinical situation of the patient, including any neurological changes

Notes

References

AAGBI. *Interhospital Transfer*. Safety Guideline. London: AAGBI, 2009

Intensive Care Society. *Guidelines for the Transport of the Critically Ill Adult*. London: Intensive Care Society, 2002

Q3 Heart-Beating Organ Donor

After brainstem testing, a patient on the neurointensive care unit is considered to be a suitable candidate for heart-beating organ donation

a) Describe the potential pathophysiological changes occurring after brain death in this patient (10 marks)

b) Outline the management of potential physiological disturbances in this patient in preparation for organ donation surgery, including clinical parameters where possible (10 marks)

Aims

A number of important factors that provide optimal organ donor conditions may be influenced by ICU doctors. By understanding the changes which may occur following brain death, appropriate interventions may be initiated.

a) Pathophysiological Changes

i) Cerebrovascular
   - Initially, massive sympathetic surge: ↑ HR, BP, CO, leading to potential myocardial damage (may be exacerbated by anaerobic metabolism and free-radical formation)
   - Manifested as arrhythmias, ST segment changes, heart blocks
   - Subsequently, loss of sympathetic control results in severe hypotension 2° to vasodilatation
   - Hypotension may also be exacerbated by hypovolaemia and myocardial dysfunction 2° to: diabetes insipidus (DI), hyperglycaemia, osmotic diuresis, or ↓ T_3 production

ii) Respiratory
   - Exacerbated by coexisting processes (e.g. sepsis, hypoxia 2° to atelectasis, fluid overload, contusions)
   - Pulmonary oedema 2° to ↑ pulmonary capillary hydrostatic pressure and left ventricular dysfunction

iii) Endocrine
   - Anterior and posterior pituitary failure
   - ↓ ADH: DI (diuresis, hypovolaemia, hyperosmolality, hypernatraemia)
   - ↓ T_3: low phosphate stores, exacerbating CVS compromise
   - ↓ cortisol: blunted stress response (↓ insulin secretion → hyperglycaemia → osmotic diuresis → metabolic acidosis → CVS compromise)

iv) Other
   - Hypothalamic failure: loss of thermoregulation, resulting in hypothermia
   - Exacerbated by peripheral vasodilatation, ↓ basal metabolic rate, and heat production
   - Coagulopathy caused by release of thromboplastin and other mediators from brain tissue

b) Optimization

i) Cerebrovascular
   - Aim for CVP 4–10mmHg, CI 2.2–2.5L/min/m², MAP 60–80mmHg, HR 60–100bpm
   - Treat hypotension initially with IV fluids
   - Consider CO monitoring, as risk of pulmonary fluid overload

- Inotropes or vasopressors for fluid-resistant hypotension:
  - vasopressin is preferred (maintains cardiac ATP, $\downarrow$ hyperosmolality, $\uparrow$ CO)
  - noradrenaline or dopamine are used if further support is required
- Correct arrhythmias (ensure electrolyte replacement is adequate)

ii) Respiratory
- Minimize FiO_2 to achieve PaO_2 >10kPa
- Protective lung ventilation (PEEP, 6mL/kg tidal volume, peak airway pressures <30cmH$_2$O)
- Note: CVP >6–8mmHg may $\uparrow$ A–a gradient

iii) Endocrine
- DI: treat with IV fluids and desmopressin (bolus or infusion)
- Hyperglycaemia is treated with an insulin infusion as per local guidelines
- IV T$_3$: $\downarrow$ inotropic requirements and $\uparrow$ cardiac stability
- High-dose methylprednisolone: $\downarrow$ inotropic requirements and $\downarrow$ extravascular lung water

iv) Other
- Maintain normothermia with fluid warmers, HME, and active body heating devices
- Correct coagulopathy with FFP, platelets, cryoprecipitate, etc.

Notes

Reference

Thomas I, Manara AR. The potential heart-beating organ donor. In: Waldmann C, Soni N, Rhodes A, eds. *Oxford Desk Reference: Critical Care*. Oxford University Press, 2008; 534–6

Q4 Hyponatraemia in Traumatic Brain Injury

a) **List the two most common causes of hyponatraemia post traumatic brain injury (2 marks)**

b) **Compare and contrast clinical and biochemical features of the above conditions (9 marks)**

c) **Outline the treatment of these conditions (9 marks)**

Aims

Hyponatraemia is a common complication post brain injury. The ability to distinguish between the causes according to clinical presentation and laboratory results has an important bearing on treatment course.

a) Causes

- Syndrome of inappropriate antidiuretic hormone (SIADH)
- Cerebral salt wasting syndrome (CSWS)

b) Clinical and Biochemical

	SIADH	CSWS
Serum Na$^+$ concentration	↓	↓
Urine Na$^+$ concentration	↑	↑
Serum osmolality	↓	↔ or ↑
Urine osmolality	↑	↑
Urine	Low volume/concentrated	High volume
Na$^+$ balance	Equal	Negative
Serum urea and creatinine	↔ or ↓	↑
Plasma volume	↑	↓
Volaemic status	Euvolaemic—no dehydration	Hypovolaemic—dehydrated
CVP	↔ or ↑	↓
Postural hypotension	No	Yes
Haematocrit	↓	↑

c) Treatment

- Progress guided by frequent U&E analysis
- i) SIADH
    - Only if symptomatic, severe hyponatraemia, or rapidly decreasing Na$^+$ levels
    - Fluid restriction: aim for serum Na$^+$ rise of 1–1.5mmol/L/day
    - Hypertonic 1.8% saline via a CVP line if very low serum Na$^+$ concentration or symptomatic
    - Demeclocycline 600–1200mg/day to inhibit the renal response of ADH
    - Oral sodium has been used
    - Consider ADH receptor antagonists (e.g. conivaptan, lixivaptan)
- ii) CSWS
    - Restoration of plasma volume and Na$^+$ concentration: initially 0.9% saline
    - Consider hypertonic saline via a CVP line

- Fludrocortisone 0.1–0.4mg/day in standard treatment-resistant cases: beware rebound hyperkalaemia

Notes

Reference

Bradshaw K, Smith M. Disorders of sodium balance after brain injury. *Continuing Education in Anaesthesia, Critical Care & Pain*, **8**: 129–33, 2008

Q5 Intracranial Pressure Measurement

a) **List signs and symptoms of a raised intracranial pressure (ICP) (7 marks)**

b) **Describe different methods of measuring ICP (7 marks)**

c) **Draw the normal and pathological waveforms for ICP (6 marks)**

Aims

When covering a neurointensive care unit, measuring and monitoring ICP levels in patients is used to aid medical and surgical interventions. You should be able to compare the relative advantages of all the techniques available, and management of raised ICP or reproduction of possible traces are other stems that may arise associated with this question.

a) Symptoms

- Headache:
  - diffuse, bifrontal, throbbing
  - worse in the morning
  - worse on lying flat/on Valsalva manoeuvre
- Visual field defects:
  - horizontal diplopia (cranial nerve VI palsy)
  - transient monocular field defects
  - narrowed visual fields, photophobia
- Non-specific:
  - dizziness, nausea and vomiting
  - tinnitus, anosmia
  - retrobulbar/back/neck pain
  - ↓ conscious level

Signs

- Bilateral papillodema: associated with macular oedema
- Cranial nerve palsies:
  - usually cranial nerve VI + horizontal nystagmus
  - occasionally bilateral
  - trochlear and occulomotor nerves
- Cushing's triad:
  - systolic hypertension
  - bradycardia
  - irregular respiration

b) ICP Measurement

i) Indirect
   Using imaging modalities (e.g. CT, MRI)
   - Sulcal effacement
   - Flattening of pituitary fossa
   - Slit-like ventricles (may also identify aetiology, i.e. tumour, bleed, trauma)
   - Orbital ultrasound (↑ CSF volume around the optic nerve is diagnostic)

ii) Direct
- Single-shot (e.g. lumbar puncture and manometry): allows assessment of CSF following procedure
- Extradural (e.g. Codmann pressure transducer)
  - ◆ Strain gauge transducer at tip of a wire which is placed either extradurally or intraparenchymally to monitor ICP
  - ◆ Inserted via small burr hole under aseptic technique. Relatively easy to insert and allows continual monitoring of ICP
  - ◆ Either air-referenced or fluid-coupled systems. Air reference avoids problem of damping traces over time, whilst fluid-filled systems have the advantage of flushing the tip of the transducer to displace debris or clot causing inaccurate measurements
  - ◆ Prone to drift and may only represent local rather than global brain tissue
- Intraventricular device (e.g. external ventricular drain)
  - ◆ Aseptic blind insertion of a tube into anterior portion of lateral ventricles via a similar approach to an ICP transducer.
  - ◆ Connected to a fluid-filled set and transduced using similar equipment to an arterial line.
  - ◆ Integrated to a system which allows fluid to be drained off into a reservoir to treat obstructive hydrocephalus
  - ◆ Represents a relatively higher infection risk compared with Codman and Camino systems

c) Waveforms of ICP Changes

i) Normal
- P1 = percussive wave: from arterial pressure transmitted from the choroid plexus.
- P2 = tidal wave: amplitude varies with brain compliance.
- P3 = dicrotic notch: caused by closure of aortic valve

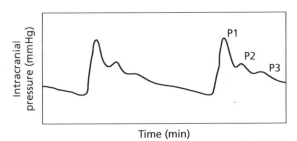

Figure 14. Normal ICP waveform

ii) Pathological
- A-wave: plateau waves of 50–100mmHg for 5–15min. Represent early brain herniation

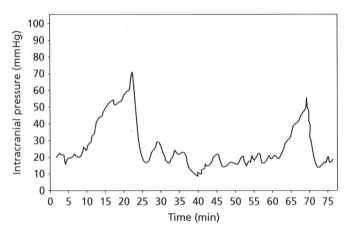

Figure 15. A-wave

- B-wave: small pressure oscillations over 30–120s. Associated with changes in respiration and gas tensions

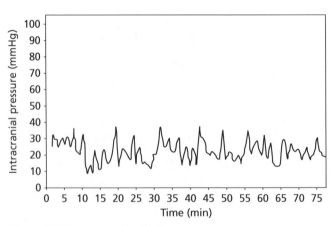

Figure 16. B-wave

- C-wave: low-amplitude changes up to five times a minute related to changes in vasomotor tone. Found in healthy and injured brains

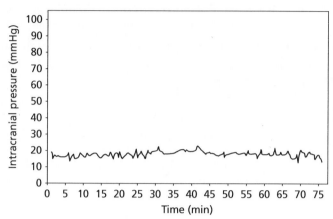

Figure 17. C-wave

Notes

....

....

....

....

....

....

....

....

....

....

....

....

Reference

Patel HC, Bouamra O, Woodford M, et al. Trends in head injury outcome from 1989 to 2003 and the effect of neurosurgical care: an observational study. *Lancet*, **366**: 1538–44, 2005

Q6 Subarachnoid Haemorrhage

A 62-year-old woman has been transported to the neurointensive care unit sedated, intubated, and ventilated following a subarachnoid haemorrhage (SAH).

a) List important complications resulting from this pathology (3 marks)

b) Outline the prevention and management of potential complications related to SAH (17 marks)

Aims

One of the main aims of critical care support of acute SAH patients is maintenance of normal physiology and prevention of further complications. It is vital to be aware of and recognize the warning signs of the deteriorating patient and be able to initiate appropriate management promptly in order to maximize the chance of successful outcome for this cohort of patients.

a) Complications

- Re-bleeding
- Cerebral vasospasm
- Hydrocephalus
- Cardiorespiratory deterioration/compromise
- Electrolyte disturbances
- Other (see below)

b) Management

i) Re-bleeding
- 15% probability on day 1; rises to 40% by the first month; mortality approximately 50%
- Thought to be associated with BP fluctuations
- Decision to occlude aneurysm based on age, comorbidities, onset time, anatomy of aneurysm, and grading
- Either surgical 'clipping' or endovascular 'coiling'
- Aim to treat all ruptured aneurysms within 72 hours
- The ISAT trial found reduced subsequent neurological complications in patients undergoing coiling compared with clipping of ruptured aneurysms. However, there were some flaws in the study, i.e. the surgical clipping group had a lower incidence of re-bleed and a higher success rate of complete aneurysmal occlusion

ii) Cerebral Vasospasm
- Most common cause of mortality; diagnosis made by CT angiography
- Peak incidence at day 7; range days 3–14; affects up to three-quarters of SAH patients
- More common in poor-grade bleeds or if large clots are present in basal cisterns

Prophylaxis
- Nimodipine PO/NG
- Magnesium: cerebral vasodilator, ↓ incidence of delayed cerebral ischaemia
- Sedation: aiming for positive fluid balance, avoiding hypotension and hyponatraemia

Treatment
- Triple H therapy:
  - hypertension using vasopressors (e.g. noradrenaline)
  - hypervolaemia using fluids
  - haemodilution to improve rheology of blood

- Other treatments include early primary balloon angioplasty and intra-arterial papaverine

iii) Hydrocephalus
- Due to either impaired reabsorption of CSF from the presence of blood in the subarachnoid space, or blood clot formation in the ventricle
- Occurs within 72 hours of the original bleed in approximately 20% of cases
- Diagnosed on CT and treated by external ventricular drainage

iv) Cardiorespiratory
- ↑ central sympathetic levels are associated with ↑ levels of sympathetic neurotransmitters and catecholamine-induced myocardial ischaemia and dysfunction
- ↑ systemic and pulmonary hypertension, pulmonary oedema, cardiogenic shock
- Cardiac arrhythmias, troponin rise, ECG and regional wall motion abnormalities
- Signs and symptoms may resolve without specific treatment, but caution with triple H therapy in severe cardiac compromise

v) Electrolyte Disturbances
- Hyponatraemia: 2° to CSW or SIADH: treat with saline or hypertonic saline infusions and/or steroids (e.g. fludrocortisone)
- Hypomagnesaemia, hypokalaemia, hypocalcaemia: corrected where required

vi) Other
- Hypothalamic dysfunction following ischaemia/infarction
- Seizures

Notes

References

Priebe HJ. Aneurysmal subarachnoid haemorrhage and the anaesthetist. *British Journal of Anaesthesia* **99**: 102–18, 2007

http://www.brainaneurysm.com/isat.html (accessed 21 April 2010)

Q7 Venous Drainage of Brain

a) **Describe the venous drainage of the cerebral circulation (6 marks)**

b) **List the risk factors for cortical vein thrombosis (CVT) (7 marks)**

c) **What clinical features are seen in cortical vein thrombosis? (7 marks)**

Aims

Despite not being an area of anatomy that you will use on a daily basis, the rare complication of cortical sinus thrombosis often requires anaesthetic input during its management. It is feasible that a question could also easily run into ICP components and the Monroe–Kellie hypothesis.

a) Venous Drainage

Broadly divided into two systems, superficial and deep

i) Superficial
   - The superficial system refers to the cortices of the cerebrum and cerebellum which drain into the superficial dural venous sinuses, whose walls are composed of dura mater, owing to their position between the two layers of the cranial dura mater
   - The superior sagittal sinus lies between the two cerebral hemispheres within the falx cerebri, draining into the left and right transverse sinuses along the border between the middle and posterior cranial fossae
   - The inferior sagittal sinus runs in the same plane but just above the corpus callosum, joining the straight sinus to anastamose with its superior neighbour
   - This point is known as the confluence of sinuses and marks the point at which the deep and superficial systems meet
   - The two transverse sinuses bend in an S-shape along the border of the tentorium cerebelli, forming the sigmoid sinuses which join with the inferior petrosal sinus to form the internal jugular vein

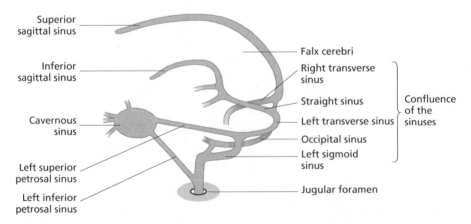

Figure 18. The venous sinuses

ii) Deep
- The deep parts of the brain drain via intra-parenchymal vessels of a traditional composition, joining behind the midbrain to form the great vein of Galen
- This vein merges with the inferior saggital sinus to form the straight sinus

b) Risk Factors for Cortical Vein Thrombosis

- Blood: stasis, low flow, dehydration, thrombocythemia
- Vessel wall trauma exposing sub-endothelial collagen, or recent surgery
- External compression (e.g. abscess (paranasal sinuses commonly implicated), tumour, or postoperative swelling/oedema)
- Systemic risk factors
  - Pregnancy (antenatal and postnatal period)
  - Hypercoagulable state (e.g. cancer, antiphospholipid syndrome, factor V Leiden deficiency, oestrogen-containing contraceptive pills, hyperhomocysteinaemia (a strong and independent risk factor for CVT, present in 27–43% of patients))
  - Inflammatory bowel disease (e.g. Crohn's disease or ulcerative colitis)
  - Haematological conditions (e.g. paroxsymal nocturnal haemoglobinuria, sickle cell disease, polycythaemia)
  - Collagen vascular diseases including SLE or Wegener's granulomatosis
  - Infection (e.g. meningitis, mastoiditis, sinusitis)
  - Any surgery to head and neck
  - Direct venous sinus trauma

c) Clinical Features

- Symptoms
  - Headache
  - Nausea and vomiting
  - Reduced level of conciousness
  - Fever
  - Diffuse encephalopathy
- Signs
  - Seizures
  - Raised ICP (e.g. papilloedema)
  - Focal neurological deficits (particularly cranial nerves V and VI)
- Rarely
  - Cranial nerve palsies
  - Cerebellar signs
  - Hemiparesis and hemisensory loss
  - Subarachnoid haemorrhage
  - Migraine + aura
  - Transient ischaemic attack
  - Tinnitus
- Cavernous sinus extension produces proptosis and periorbital oedema
- Symptoms are usually unilateral but can extend to become bilateral. This is thought to represent extension of the thrombus to the contralateral side

Notes

Reference

http://www.uptodate.com/patients/content/topic.do?topicKey=~jlSOjZvXWJczdq6 (accessed 14 May 2010)

Chapter 5: **Paediatric Anaesthesia**

Q1 Bleeding Tonsil

The ENT surgeons wish to return to theatre with a 4-year-old girl who is bleeding from the mouth 5 hours post-tonsillectomy. She weighs 16kg.

a) **Outline the important factors in preoperative assessment of this child (7 marks)**

b) **Describe a safe induction technique in this case (7 marks)**

c) **How can postoperative pain, nausea, and vomiting be minimized? (6 marks)**

Aims

This is an ENT and anaesthetic paediatric emergency. It is a common topic in the examination as it tests the candidate's knowledge of and ability in paediatric assessment, resuscitation, and emergency induction of a potentially life-threatening condition.

a) Preoperative Assessment

- Visit the child and parents on the ward to initiate resuscitation, establish rapport, obtain a history, perform an examination and investigations, and gain consent
- History: timing of events, look at previous anaesthetic chart (doses, ETT size, and technique)
- Examination
  - Assess for signs of hypovolaemia (e.g. HR, capillary refill time, mental status, skin turgor)
  - Blood loss may be masked, and therefore greater than estimated, by swallowed blood and the maintenance of physiological reserve
  - There may be residual anaesthetic status
- Investigations: obtain IV access (if not done already) and take blood samples for FBC, clotting, U&E, and cross-match
- Resuscitation: 320mL (20mL/kg) bolus of crystalloid (e.g. Hartmann's solution) and observe physiological parameters for response. Repeat if required. Consider packed red cells if no improvement

b) Induction

- Senior anaesthetist should be present for this case
- Use technique most familiar with. Both IV RSI in the supine position and inhalational induction in a head-down left lateral position are advocated. However, these techniques should not be used if they are unfamiliar
- High risk of regurgitation and aspiration due to a full stomach 2° to swallowed blood; therefore RSI, if IV. Ensure preoxygenation >3min and cricoid pressure
- Potentially challenging as active bleeding may be present in an uncooperative child. The presence of blood clots may also obscure anatomy at laryngoscopy
- Two suction devices under pillow (one may become blocked by clots)
- IV induction: thiopental 80mg (5mg/kg) and suxamethonium 16mg (1mg/kg). Care with induction agents in hypovolaemia
- Intubate with a predicted # 5.0 south-facing RAE OETT and check for bilateral air entry. May require a smaller tube size if used in previous anaesthetic or airway oedema is present from prior instrumentation
- Spontaneous ventilation or IPPV, and maintenance: O_2 + air or N_2O + volatile agent
- Surgeons scrubbed and ready to operate

c) Analgesia and Anti-emesis

i) Analgesia
  - Intraoperative opiate: IV fentanyl 16–50mcg (1–4mcg/kg). Caution with excess opioid administration in a potentially hypovolaemic child having a second anaesthetic within 24 hours
  - Postoperative: PO paracetamol 320mg (20mg/kg), and oramorph 3.2–6.4mg (0.2–0.4 mg/kg)

ii) Anti-emesis
  - Empty stomach post procedure with wide-bore orogastric tube
  - IV crystalloid resuscitation and maintenance fluid rate of 52mL/hour
  - Consider anti-emetics (e.g. IV ondansetron 2.4mg (0.15mg/kg) and IV dexamethasone 2.4mg (0.15mg/kg)), although they may mask ongoing tonsil bleeding into the stomach postoperatively

Notes

Reference

Dickson E. Bleeding tonsil or adenoids. In: Doyle E, ed. *Paediatric Anaesthesia*. Oxford Specialist Handbooks in Anaesthesia. Oxford University Press, 2007; 416

Q2 Caudal Anaesthesia

a) **For which surgical procedures would a caudal block provide adequate analgesia in paediatric patients? (5 marks)**

b) **Describe the technique of caudal injection, including anatomical landmarks and relevant drug doses (11 marks)**

c) **List complications of this technique (4 marks)**

Aims

Paediatric caudal anaesthesia provides a useful opioid-sparing analgesic adjunct. Candidates should be familiar with both the technique and potential complications which may be discussed during consent

a) Surgical Procedures

i) General Surgery
   - Inguinal hernia repair
   - Any surgery on the distal GI tract (i.e. rectum or anus)
   - Orchidopexy, circumcision (cross-over with urology)

ii) Urology
   - Hypospadias repair
   - Orchidopexy, circumcision (cross-over with general surgery)

iii) Other
   - Lower limb plastic or orthopaedic surgery

b) Technique

- Standard anaesthetic history and examination, and procedural consent (from parents)
  - S   Sterile technique
  - L   Light source
  - I   IV access
  - M   Monitoring
  - R   Resuscitation equipment
  - A   Assistant trained in regional and general anaesthesia
  - G   Ability to convert to GA (not applicable here)
- Left lateral position is commonly used
- Hips and knees are flexed to 90°: optimal for palpation of the sacral hiatus
- Confirm the boundaries of the sacral hiatus: an equilateral triangle is formed from lines joining the sacral cornua inferiorly and the apex at the body of S4 superiorly
- Identify the puncture site and clean with 0.5% chlorhexidine. Allow evaporation before attempting the block
- A blunt short-bevel needle is inserted through the skin at a 45° angle until a click is felt as the sacrococcygeal membrane is punctured. At this point the needle is directed in a cephalad direction along the long axis of the sacral canal
- A 20G or 22G IV cannula can also be used; once the membrane is pierced, the needle can be withdrawn and the blunt cannula advanced, reducing the chance of accidental dural puncture. The cannula should advance easily; any resistance should prompt re-insertion
- ECG monitoring is mandatory to exclude intravascular injection of LA

- Confirmation is achieved by:
  - aspiration to exclude subarachnoid or intravascular placement
  - ease of injection—should be virtually no resistance
  - ultrasound may confirm injection of LA into the epidural space
- Drugs
  - Armitage regimen using 0.25% bupivacaine with volume calculated according to the level of block required (maximum 20mL total volume LA):
  - lumbosacral 0.5mL/kg
  - thoracolumbar 1mL/kg
  - mid-thoracic 1.25ml/kg
  - additives to improve duration and quality of block: clonidine 1–2mcg/kg or ketamine (preservative free) 0.5mg/kg

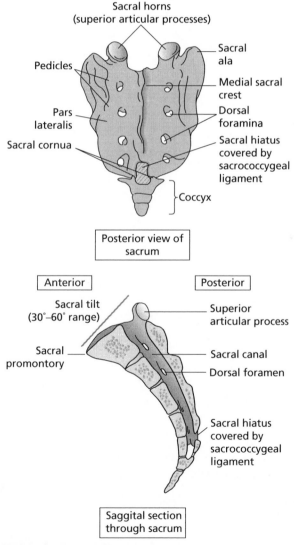

Figure 19. The sacrum

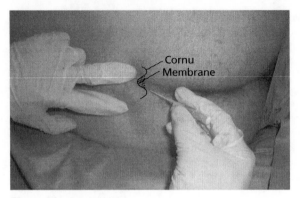

Figure 20. Caudal block

c) Complications

- Intravascular or intraosseous injection
- Dural puncture
- Motor block
- Urinary retention
- Perforation of the rectum
- Subcutaneous injection
- Haematoma
- Failure

Notes

Q3 Foreign Body Aspiration

You are asked to assess a 2-year-old girl in the Emergency Department with a persistent and worsening cough whose mother reports an episode of choking following playing with plastic beads 2 days ago. On examination, she is apyrexial with bilateral air entry and no wheeze on auscultation. Clinically, you suspect a foreign body aspiration.

a) List differential diagnoses for this presentation (5 marks)

b) What would you expect to find on a chest radiograph? (4 marks)

c) How would you anaesthetise this child for bronchoscopy under GA? (11 marks)

Aims

Candidates must recognize the need for an inhalational induction and maintenance of spontaneous ventilation for this procedure. Familiarity with types of bronchoscopy equipment and their relative merits is important.

a) Differential Diagnoses

- Foreign body
- Croup
- Epiglottitis
- Whooping cough/diphtheria
- Lower respiratory tract infection
- Asthma
- URTI
- Bronchiolitis (rarely at this age)

b) Investigations

Should be minimal to avoid upsetting the child
- CXR may be normal
- May rarely see foreign body if very radio-opaque
- Lobar collapse, mediastinal shift
- End-expiratory film or fluoroscopy screening: hyperinflation during expiration if child is cooperative, or unilateral emphysema

c) Anaesthesia

- Preassessment: standard history, examination, and consent from parents
    - if no evidence of respiratory distress, consider waiting until the child is starved
    - avoid distress in the child, potentially exacerbating further obstruction
- Two experienced anaesthetists for induction (at least one consultant experienced with paediatric patients)
- Experienced assistant, emergency equipment and drugs, anaesthetic machine check
- Recommended technique is inhalational induction: O_2 and sevoflurane with emphasis on maintenance of spontaneous ventilation
- Once depth of anaesthesia is adequate:
    - obtain IV access and give an anti-sialogogue (e.g. atropine 20mcg/kg) to minimize secretions

- ♦ administer lidocaine spray (max. 4mg/kg) to the vocal cords and larynx to prevent coughing prior to airway instrumentation with bronchoscope
- Position: supine with neck extension using inter-scapular support (e.g. IV fluid bag)
- Use a Storz bronchoscope with a side-arm attachment for Ayre's T-piece to provide O_2, anaesthesia, and ventilation
- Usual technique is gentle IPPV as spontaneous ventilation may be hard to maintain with potential coughing or breath-holding
- Consider a background propofol infusion if spontaneous ventilation technique used to maintain adequate depth of anaesthesia
- Administer IV dexamethasone 0.25mg/kg to minimize airway tissue swelling and oedema
- If significant airway swelling, respiratory distress, or trauma 2° to procedure, intubate and ventilate, and transfer to ICU
- Humidified O_2, physiotherapy, regular dexamethasone; may require antibiotics

Notes

Reference

Weir PM. Foreign body aspiration. In: Stoddart PA, Lauder GR, eds. *Problems in Anaesthesia: Paediatric Anaesthesia*. London: Martin Dunitz, 2004; 163–6

Q4 Inhalational Induction

a) List the indications (3 marks) and contraindications (3 marks) for inhalational induction of anaesthesia in a child

b) Describe a technique for performing paediatric inhalational induction (14 marks)

Aims

Children can be technically difficult to cannulate, whether because of lack of cooperation or 'fat pads' on the hands. Inhalational induction is a common technique, but it is not without potential problems to be aware of.

a) Indications and Contraindications

i) Indications
   - Parental or patient request (e.g. 2° to needle phobia or repeat procedures)
   - Poor or difficult venous access (e.g. infant with chubby hands and feet)
   - Potentially difficult airway or anticipated difficult manual ventilation (e.g. epiglottitis)
   - Presence of foreign body in the larynx or tracheobronchial tree

ii) Contraindications
   - Uncooperative patient or parent (difficult at 'ethically tricky' age range; need to assess the urgency of the procedure and postpone with adequate preparation)
   - Severe cardiovascular compromise (e.g. severe hypovolaemia, fixed cardiac output state, cardiac failure, right-to-left shunt)
   - Malignant hyperthermia

b) Technique

- Pre-assessment: full explanation to parents of technique, with consent for inhalational induction. Appropriate explanation to child depending on age
- Emergency drugs (suxamethonium 1–2mg/kg and atropine 10–20mcg/kg) are prepared
- Decide whether the child will cooperate with induction lying on trolley or sitting across parent's lap
- If sitting across parent's lap, ensure correct position of parent and child prior to starting to allow for ease and rapidity of transfer of child when unconscious
- If the child will cooperate, place a pulse oximeter probe on the finger or toe
- Some anaesthetists use scented pens or face masks to hide the odour of anaesthetic agents
- Some anaesthetists use a mask; others remove the mask and cup their hand around the tubing close to the mouth and nose in younger children
- Parents should be warned of abnormal movements during induction
- Inhalational induction is with a volatile agent such as sevoflurane (halothane is still used in some centres) and O_2 with air or N_2O according to preference
- Sevoflurane concentration may be ↑ incrementally or commenced at high levels; halothane should be ↑ incrementally to avoid distress
- Once the child is unconscious, he/she is transferred whilst supporting the head, neck, and body to the trolley, and the parents are escorted from the theatre suite by the paediatric nurse
- At this point, if not already done, standard AAGBI monitoring (pulse oximetry, NIBP, ECG) is instituted

- The airway is supported (with oropharyngeal airway if required), the child is ventilated if appropriate, and venous access is obtained once the child is at a sufficiently deep level of anaesthesia
- Remember to ↓ the concentration of inspired volatile agent once adequately anaesthetised to avoid subsequent cardiovascular or respiratory depression
- Upon obtaining venous access, appropriate drugs may be administered, and airway devices inserted (e.g. LMA or ETT)

Notes

....

....

....

....

....

....

....

....

....

....

....

....

Reference

Eccles P. Inhalational induction of anaesthesia. In: Doyle E, ed. *Paediatric Anaesthesia*. Oxford Specialist Handbooks in Anaesthesia. Oxford University Press, 2007; 64–5

Q5 Paediatric Murmur

Whilst pre-assessing a 2 year old child for grommet insertion, a previously undiscovered heart murmur is auscultated.

a) **What factors allow clinicians to distinguish between innocent and pathological murmurs in children? (11 marks)**

b) **List the actions to take if a murmur is discovered, include investigations where relevant (9 marks)**

Aims

It is not unusual to encounter children with murmurs in pre-assessment. Thus it is important to assess those that possess a clinical relevance, either allowing surgery to proceed or referring for further investigations.

a) Factors

  i) Innocent Murmur
   - Normal growth and exercise tolerance, history asymptomatic of typical cardiac symptoms (e.g. shortness of breath, cyanosis)
   - On examination
     - Normal heart sounds
     - Soft, early, or blowing systolic murmur (usually from pulmonary outflow, heard over the second left intercostal space)
     - Short 'buzzing' murmur (usually from left side of heart, heard over the fourth left intercostal space)
     - No radiation of murmur
     - Venous hum
     - Presence of fever (due to $\uparrow$ cardiac output)

  ii) Pathological Murmur
   - Evidence of congenital heart disease from notes, parents, or in family
   - History of failure to thrive, poor feeding, reduced exercise tolerance, cyanosis (e.g. when crying)
   - On examination
     - Abnormal added heart sounds (e.g. 'click')
     - Pansystolic, ejection systolic, or diastolic loud murmur
     - Sternal heave
     - Parasternal thrill
     - Abnormal peripheral pulses (e.g. weakened femoral arterial pulsation)

b) Innocent Murmur

- Options will depend on local guidelines: a preoperative ECG should be performed
- It is important to consider that both aortic stenosis and hypertrophic cardiomyopathy may present as an 'innocent' murmur with few symptoms. Further investigations (e.g. ECG, CXR, echo) should be performed if more sinister pathologies are suspected
- If there is anything suspicious in the history, examination, or ECG, referral to a paediatric cardiologist is warranted

i) Options

Proceed with Surgery

- Antibiotic prophylaxis is currently administered according to local guidelines for surgery likely to cause bacteraemia (e.g. dental) and is *unlikely* to be required for grommet insertion
- Organize postoperative investigations to identify and document murmur for future cases

Delay Surgery for Investigations

- Evaluate the urgency of the operation. If elective, as in this case, postpone the operation until the child has been fully investigated
- Referral to a paediatric cardiologist preoperatively with the ECG for expert opinion and echocardiogram
- Include a chest radiograph if evidence of respiratory symptoms
- Documentation in notes and parental education will be required

Notes

Reference

Eccles P. Heart murmurs. In: Doyle, E ed. *Paediatric Anaesthesia.* Oxford Specialist Handbooks in Anaesthesia. Oxford University Press, 2007; 70–1

Q6 **Paediatric PONV**

a) **List important risk factors for postoperative nausea and vomiting (PONV) in children (12 marks)**

b) **What pharmacological and non-pharmacological strategies exist to minimize or prevent postoperative nausea and vomiting in children? (8 marks)**

Aims

PONV can have significant implications on a surgical patient's postoperative care. Whilst being undesirable and distressing from a patient and parent perspective, logistical issues are also involved, including bed management and the cost of overnight admission. All of these factors must be integrated into your answer when justifying the aims to reduce this phenomenon.

a) Risk Factors

i) Patient-Related
   * Age: likelihood of PONV increases >3 years old and increases into adolescence
   * Past history of PONV in previous operations
   * Family history of PONV
   * History of travel or motion sickness
   * Females > males (only in adolescence after puberty)

ii) Surgery-Related
   * Procedure-related
   * High-risk include:
     ◆ ophthalmic surgery (e.g. strabismus correction): incidence of 50–90%
     ◆ ENT (adenotonsillectomy, middle and external ear surgery)
     ◆ gynaecological (adolescents)
     ◆ laparoscopic surgery
   * Duration-related (>30min operating time)

iii) Anaesthetic-Related
   * Opioid use: long-acting > short-acting, postoperative > intraoperative
   * Choice of anaesthesia: use of volatiles or anticholinesterases (less than adults) increases the risk. The link between PONV and N_2O is not proven
   * Administration of intraoperative IV fluids reduces PONV risk, but mandatory oral fluid intake prior to day-case discharge increases PONV risk

b) Prevention of PONV

   * Recognition of the patient at high-risk for PONV because of the above factors is the key to success

i) Pharmacological
   * Children at increased risk of PONV: IV ondansetron 0.15mg/kg at induction up to 4mg
   * Children at very high risk: IV ondansetron 0.15mg/kg prophylactic *and* IV dexamethasone 0.15mg/kg
   * Use non-opioid analgesics where possible (e.g. paracetamol, NSAIDs)
   * Use short-acting opioids (e.g. fentanyl) if required
   * Consider the use of total IV anaesthesia in extremely high-risk patients (contraindicated in children <3 years old)

ii) Non-Pharmacological
- Intraoperative intravenous fluid therapy
- Regional techniques (e.g. caudals) are opioid-avoiding
- A meta-analysis has shown that stimulation of the P6 acupuncture point is equally as effective as anti-emetic drugs in preventing PONV

Notes

_____

_____

_____

_____

_____

_____

_____

_____

_____

_____

_____

Reference

APAGBI. *Guidelines on the Prevention of Post-operative Vomiting in Children.* London: APAGBI, 2009

Q7 Prematurity

A 2-month-old boy presents for elective repair of a left inguinal hernia. He was born at 31 weeks weighing 1.1kg and required ventilation for 9 days on SCBU. He was eventually discharged home after 5 weeks in hospital. He now weighs 2.5kg.

a) List the implications of prematurity which may affect anaesthesia in this baby (9 marks)

b) Which anaesthetic technique may be used? (7 marks)

c) Outline important factors in postoperative care for this baby (4 marks)

Aims

During on-call duties and paediatric modules, candidates may be involved in anaesthetising premature babies. These patients present a unique set of issues which can be challenging cases for a variety of reasons, and awareness of this can help plan for safe anaesthetic technique.

a) Prematurity

i) Respiratory and Airway
  - Chronic respiratory disease: airway irritability, decreased compliance, V/Q mismatch, increased work of breathing
  - Postoperative respiratory apnoea, i.e. apnoea >15s without bradycardia, or <15s with bradycardia for 12–24 hours post-GA
  - Subglottic or tracheal stenosis, tracheomalacia

ii) Cardiovascular
  - Patent ductus arteriosus
  - Prone to bradycardias

iii) Neurological
  - Intraventricular haemorrhage, hydrocephalus
  - Developmental delay, cerebral palsy risk, hypoxic brain injury, seizures

iv) Other
  - Poor nutrition
  - Anaemia or clotting abnormalities
  - Poor venous access due to multiple previous cannulations
  - If significant physiological problems exist, discuss with surgeon re delaying procedure until older. The procedure should be performed in a tertiary paediatric centre with PICU support

b) Anaesthetic Techniques

i) Preoperative Assessment
  - Anaesthetic history (including details of any perinatal complications), examination, and parental consent
  - Avoid prolonged fasting (risk of hypoglycaemia and dehydration): follow local fasting guidelines and consider preoperative IV fluid infusion
  - Two paediatric anaesthetists for this case

ii) Intraoperative
  - If severely O_2 dependent, consider an awake spinal block ± sedation. Otherwise general anaesthesia

- ◆ Tracheal intubation and mechanical ventilation: greater control over airway and gas exchange
- ◆ O_2, air, and volatile agent maintenance (e.g. sevoflurane)
- Insert an NG tube to empty and deflate the stomach
- Care with opioids: sensitivity and ↑ risk of postoperative apnoea
- Consider a caudal block or LA infiltration by the surgeon
- PR paracetamol 50mg (20mg/kg)
- Maintain normothermia with underbody heating and warmed IV fluids
- Perioperative IV fluid therapy, ensuring maintenance of normoglycaemia

c) Postoperative Care

- If particularly high-risk case, transfer to HDU or PICU
- High risk of postoperative respiratory apnoea ± bradycardias for up to 24 hours post-GA. Therefore respiratory monitoring is mandatory: SpO_2, RR, HR, and apnoea alarming
- Analgesia: PO paracetamol and codeine should be sufficient if LA/RA is successful
- Encourage return to feeding as soon as possible: postoperative IV fluid regimen according to local guidelines is initiated if not feeding or vomiting

Notes

Q8 Premedication

During pre-assessment of a 5-year-old girl with delayed educational development for grommet insertion, her mother asks whether a 'premed' would be possible prior to anaesthesia.

a) List the indications for premedication in children (5 marks)

b) Outline advantages and disadvantages of commonly used sedatives and analgesics; where possible include recommended dosage (15 marks)

Aims

This SAQ tests premedication pharmacology. It emphasizes the importance of the preoperative visit, clear explanations of procedure, and potential side effects of drugs.

a) Indications for Premedication

- Anxiolysis
- Analgesia: either pre-emptive or for patients in pain preoperatively
- Promotion of amnesia
- Reduction of secretions
- Reduction of volume and pH of gastric contents
- Reduction of postoperative nausea and vomiting
- Reduction of vagal reflexes to intubation
- Specific indications, i.e. antibiotics or anticoagulants

b) Commonly Used Agents

i) Benzodiazepines
  - Midazolam is the main agent used in practice in the UK
  - Good anxiolytic and amnesic effects
  - Reduces the incidence of postoperative behavioural disturbances
  - Minimal effects on recovery and discharge times when used in doses of 0.5mg/kg; onset within 15–20min
  - Administration via a variety of routes is possible
    - Oral 0.5mg/kg up to 20mg: unpleasant to taste; can dilute with paracetamol or fruit squash
    - Nasal 0.2 mg/kg: faster onset, less patient cooperation required. Associated with an unpleasant burning sensation. A high-concentration low-pH solution is available at some hospitals
    - Sublingual 0.2mg/kg: rapid onset but requires patient compliance
    - IV 0.1–0.2mg/kg: requires cannula insertion, very fast onset
  - Anti-emetic effect associated with benzodiazepines
  - Can have the opposite effect in some children and cause hyperactivity

ii) Ketamine
  - Variety of routes of administration possible (IV, IM, PO, nasal, sublingual)
  - Dose 5–8mg/kg PO
  - Analgesic, anxiolytic, sedative, and bronchodilatory effect
  - Sympathetic stimulation associated with increased secretions
  - Used where midazolam may be ineffective
  - Hallucinations and emergence reactions are common (may be counteracted by benzodiazepine adjunct)

- Dystonic movements are common
- May prolong hospital stay and delay discharge; therefore less suitable for day surgery

iii) Fentanyl
- Strong OP-3 agonist; available as a lollipop
- Dose of 15–20mcg/kg associated with sedation and anxiolysis
- Good analgesic effect within 15–20min
- Associated with nausea, vomiting, itching, and respiratory depression

iv) Other Options
- Paracetamol 20mg/kg
- Ibuprofen 10mg/kg
- Clonidine 4mcg/kg: unsuitable for day surgery because of prolonged sedation effects

Notes

References

Brennan LJ, Prabhu AJ. Paediatric day-case anaesthesia. *Continuing Education in Anaesthesia, Critical Care & Pain*, **8**: 134–8, 2003

Tan L, Meakin GH. Anaesthesia for the uncooperative child. *Continuing Education in Anaesthesia, Critical Care & Pain*, **10**: 48–52, 2010

Q9 Pyloric Stenosis

A 6-week-old child presents to the paediatricians with a one-week history of projectile vomiting and weight loss. There is visible peristalsis followed by a projectile vomit after a test feed and an epigastric mass can be palpated.

The blood results demonstrated:

Na$^+$ 139mmol/L	pH 7.51
K$^+$ 2.9mmol/L	Po$_2$ 8.0
Urea 7mmol/L	Pco$_2$ 5.1
Cr 42µmol/L	HCO$_3^-$ 32
Cl$^-$ 90mmol/L	Base excess +5

a) What is the condition and how frequently does it occur? (6 marks)

b) Outline preoperative preparation of this case prior to surgery (7 marks)

c) Discuss the perioperative anaesthetic management of this case (7 marks)

Aims

Candidates must insist on preoperative resuscitation prior to anaesthesia and should be aware of the different induction options in this case.

a) Condition

- Pyloric stenosis: a congenital hypertrophy of the circular and longitudinal muscle around the pylorus of the stomach with oedema of the pyloric mucosa
- Passage of gastric contents through to the duodenum is blocked and classically the baby has non-bilious projectile vomiting
- Frequency is 1 in 400 live births and commonly affects first-born male infants and premature infants. It is 15 times more likely in children of parents who were themselves affected
- There is controversy about the need to transfer patients to a major hospital with a paediatric intensive care unit
- The general rule is that these cases should only be treated outside specialist centres if there is a reasonable caseload of children requiring surgery in this age group and the surgeon, anaesthetist, and ward and theatre staff all have appropriate training and experience

b) Preoperative Preparation

- Standard anaesthetic history, examination, parental consent, and read the notes
- If premature (i.e. <37 weeks post-conceptual age), consider transfer to a specialist centre (child more prone to postoperative hypoglycaemia and apnoeic spells)
- Associated abnormalities may include Pierre–Robin sequence (potentially difficult airway management)
- Keep child nil by mouth, insert cannula, and give IV fluids
- Insert NG tube, put it on free drainage, and regularly aspirate it
- Assess for dehydration (anterior fontanelle, eyes sunken, delayed capillary refill)
- If severely dehydrated, give initial bolus of 20mL/kg 0.9% saline and re-assess
- Correct dehydration, metabolic alkalosis, and electrolyte abnormalities over 24 hours using 0.9% saline with K$^+$ supplementation where indicated

- Obtain informed consent from parents
- Surgery should be performed electively when fluid and electrolyte abnormalities are corrected

c) Perioperative Management

- Connect monitoring in warmed anaesthetic room or in the operating theatre itself, avoiding the need to disconnect from one machine and transfer the baby
- Ensure thorough gastric emptying with 'four-quadrant' aspiration of the NG tube
- Consider an anti-sialogogue, e.g. IV atropine 20mcg/kg
- There is considerable debate regarding the use of RSI and cricoid pressure for this procedure if gastric emptying is thorough
- Options include the following
  - RSI: thiopental 4–5mg/kg and suxamethonium 2mg/kg
  - Some anaesthetists prefer a gaseous induction with sevoflurane and O_2 followed by a muscle relaxant (e.g. atracurium 0.5mg/kg)
- Intubate with an uncuffed ETT size 3.0 or 3.5
- IPPV is the usual technique: maintenance is with air, oxygen, and a volatile agent
- Monitor and maintain temperature using underbody heating and warmed IV fluids
- Antibiotics are administered according to local guidelines
- Analgesia: 30mg/kg paracetamol PR and local infiltration by the surgeon, e.g. 0.8ml/kg of 0.25% bupivacaine
- Reverse muscle relaxation: neostigmine 50mcg/kg and glycopyrollate 10mcg/kg
- Extubate in the left lateral position when the baby is fully awake
- Postoperative analgesia: PO paracetamol 15mg/kg up to 60mg/kg per 24 hours
- Monitoring should include apnoea monitoring for the first 12 hours
- Postoperative feeding is restarted according to local unit guidelines

Notes

Reference

Carr AS. Anaesthetic management for pyloromyotomy in a district general hospital. In: Stoddart PA, Lauder GR, eds. *Problems in Anaesthesia: Paediatric Anaesthesia*. London: Martin Dunitz, 2004; 13–18

Q10 Stridor

You are called to assess a 2-year-old girl in the Emergency Department whose mother describes a four-day history of malaise, low-grade pyrexia, and worsening cough. She has now developed stridor and is becoming increasingly agitated.

a) List the differential diagnoses of acute stridor in this child (4 marks)

b) What would be the indications for airway intervention in this situation? (2 marks)

c) Following diagnosis, describe your management plan for this child (14 marks)

Aims

This is a paediatric emergency warranting attendance and management by senior clinicians. Emphasis is placed on not upsetting the child and appropriate airway management.

a) Differential Diagnoses

- Croup (laryngotracheobronchitis)
- Acute epiglottitis (*Haemophilis influenza B*)
- Laryngotracheitis
- Acute pharyngitis
- Acute tonsillitis
- Retropharyngeal abscess
- Diphtheria

b) Airway Intervention

- Worsening airway obstruction
- Evidence of deteriorating respiratory function: tachypnoea, use of accessory respiratory muscles, low saturations despite supplementary O_2, agitation (2° to hypoxia)

c) Initial Management

- Senior involvement should be present i.e. two anaesthetists and an ENT consultant
- Airway: assess obstruction. Is intubation warranted imminently?
- Breathing: look for signs of respiratory distress, quiet breathing, not talking
- Administer high-flow O_2 and initiate SpO_2 monitoring
- Circulation
- Consider nebulized adrenaline 3–5mL of 1:1000 (max. 5mg): requires ECG monitoring during administration
- Avoid any actions which may upset child and worsen obstruction; if IV cannulation is essential, use topical LA cream
- Transfer to theatre with appropriate monitoring and airway equipment
- Inhalational induction initially in the sitting position with O_2 and sevoflurane; may take some time. Gradually change to supine position; aim to maintain spontaneous ventilation
- Low-level CPAP may improve airway obstruction
- Ensure depth of anaesthesia is adequate prior to IV access attempt and intubation; have a range of ETT sizes available
- Secure IV access once deep and administer an anti-sialogogue, e.g. IV atropine 20mcg/kg
- Intubate with ENT surgeon on standby for tracheostomy if failure to secure airway (anatomy may be grossly distorted)

- If intubation is easy, change the oral ETT for a nasal ETT (easier for PICU care)
- Once stable, paralyse and sedate for transfer to PICU for further care:
  - CXR
  - NG tube
  - IV fluids
  - Blood cultures then IV antibiotics according to local guidelines

Notes

Reference

Dickson E. Stridor. In: Doyle E, ed. *Paediatric Anaesthesia*, Oxford Specialist Handbooks in Anaesthesia. Oxford University Press, 2007; 420–2

Part 2 **Critical Care Medicine**

Q1 Abdominal Compartment Syndrome

A 57-year-old man on ICU has developed hypotension, oliguria, and high peak airway pressures 12 hours post Hartmann's procedure for caecal perforation. You suspect that he may be developing abdominal compartment syndrome (ACS).

a) Define intra-abdominal hypertension and ACS (2 marks)

b) What methods exist for measuring intra-abdominal pressures? (6 marks)

c) Describe the management of a patient with suspected ACS (12 marks)

Aims

Candidates should be able to connect the clinical deterioration of a post-laparotomy patient with a diagnosis of ACS, despite a plethora of potential reasons for the complications listed.

a) Definitions

- Normal intra-abdominal pressure in ICU patients: 5–7mmHg
- Intra-abdominal hypertension: >12mmHg continuously or on repeated measurements
- ACS: >20mmHg with associated single- or multi-organ dysfunction

b) Measuring IAP

- Indirectly: transduction most commonly via a urinary bladder catheter to measure intravesical pressure
  - 100mL of sterile saline is introduced into the bladder and the drainage bag is re-connected and cross-clamped
  - A 16G needle is connected to a manometer or pressure transducer and introduced via the culture port site of the catheter
  - The patient remains supine and the zero point is at the symphysis pubis
- Directly: via the introduction of a needle into the abdomen (e.g. during laparoscopy)

c) Management of ACS

- Mortality figures are >40%, so prompt decisive treatment is imperative (if left untreated, mortality is much higher)
- The priority is to optimize the patient's physiological and metabolic status, and restore and improve vital organ function, including:
  - aggressive IV fluid resuscitation
  - inotropes and/or vasopressors
- Optimal ventilator settings to deliver adequate ventilation without risk of acute lung injury
- Adequate sedation, analgesia, and muscle relaxation to avoid coughing, straining, or peritoneal irritation
- Avoid the prone position
- Consider renal replacement therapy (if severe acidosis or gross electrolyte balance)
- Gastric decompression and the use of prokinetics
- Drainage of any intra-abdominal collections
- Surgical decompression and laparostomy formation
- Ultimately the definitive treatment's success is indicated by an improvement in physiological parameters, depending on the initial cause
- Use of a negative-pressure suction dressing is common postoperatively

- Complications include management of an open abdomen on ICU, fluid loss, skin care, and the potential for fistula formation

Notes

....

....

....

....

....

....

....

....

....

....

....

....

References

Bersten D, Soni N. *Oh's Intensive Care Manual* (6th edn). Oxford: Butterworth Heinemann Elsevier, 2009; 502–3

Hopkins D, Gemmill LW. Intra-abdominal hypertension and the abdominal compartment syndrome. *Continuing Education in Anaesthesia, Critical Care & Pain*, **1**: 56–9, 2001

Waldmann C, Soni N, Rhodes A (eds). *Oxford Desk Reference: Critical Care*. Oxford University Press, 2008: 344–5

Q2 Acute Renal Failure

a) What are the different indications for renal replacement therapy? (5 marks)

b) Compare modes of renal replacement available in ICU (9 marks)

c) List potential complications of renal replacement therapy (6 marks)

Aims

All candidates should have experience of initiating and managing patients for renal replacement therapy and should be able to recognize potential pitfalls. This topic is also popular in the SOE section.

a) Indications

- Renal triggers
  - Oliguria or anuria
  - Severe fluid overload and pulmonary oedema 2° to oliguria or anuria
  - Hyperkalaemia
  - Metabolic acidosis
  - Clinically symptomatic uraemia
- Improved clearance
  - Poisoning or overdose (e.g. salicylates)
  - Temperature management (e.g. malignant hyperthermia)
- Systemic pathology
  - Multi-organ dysfunction syndrome
  - Sepsis: thought to clear cytokines but no long-term survival trend exists
  - Non-renal fluid overload (i.e. heart failure)

b) Modes of Renal Support

Classified according to the following.

i) Continuous vs. Intermittent Techniques
   - A recent meta-analysis showed no difference in renal or overall outcome. Continuous is the default strategy in most units

ii) Source of Pressure Gradient
   - Arteriovenous or venovenous
     - Venovenous requires external roller-pumps to generate a pressure gradient

iii) Process of Solute Removal
   - Haemofiltration (e.g. continuous venovenous haemofiltration)
     - Clearance of solutes is via convection
     - Rate of solute removal is determined by blood flow, transmembrane pressure gradient, and membrane coefficient (pore size/permeability)
     - Filtrate removal is balanced by the addition of a solution to maintain volume
   - Haemodialysis (e.g. continuous venovenous haemodialysis)
     - Diffusion down a concentration gradient created by a dialysate across a selectively permeable membrane
     - Continuous venovenous mode with a low permeability membrane; clearance is via diffusion and limited to small molecules
     - No fluid is added to the filtrate after diffusion

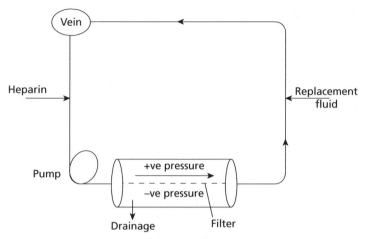

Figure 21. Continuous venovenous haemofiltration

- Combination (e.g. continuous venovenous haemodiafiltration)
  - Continuous venovenous mode with a high permeability membrane; counter-current dialysate is used
  - Solute removal is via diffusion and convection; fluid replacement is required to maintain plasma volume

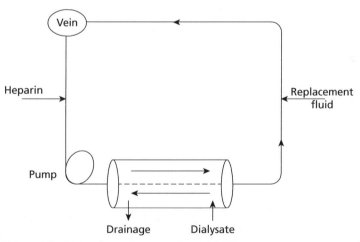

Figure 22. Continuous venovenous haemodiafiltration

iv) Dose of Renal Replacement Therapy
- Current research suggests that a rate of 20–25mL/kg is adequate. Higher rates of clearance (35–40mL/kg) confer no benefit and may be associated with risk

c) Complications

- Due to the cannula:
  - haemorrhage
  - infection
  - distal limb vascular occlusion (e.g. ischaemia, thrombosis)
- Due to the filter:
  - hypovolaemia, fluid overload, anaemia
  - electrolyte abnormalities, disequilibrium syndrome
  - air embolism
  - hypothermia
  - haemolysis
  - thrombosis
  - anaphylactoid reactions (seen in patients on ACE inhibitors using AN69 membranes)
- Due to anticoagulation:
  - haemorrhage
  - thrombocytopenia (including heparin-induced)

Notes

References

Bellomo R, Cass A, Cole L, *et al.* (2009). Intensity of continuous renal-replacement therapy in critically ill patients. *New England Journal of Medicine*, **361**: 1627–38

Ronco C, Ricci Z. In: Waldmann C, Soni N, Rhodes A, eds. *Oxford Desk Reference: Critical Care.* Oxford University Press, 2008; 68–9

Short A. Haemodialysis. In: Waldmann C, Soni N, Rhodes A, eds. *Oxford Desk Reference: Critical Care.* Oxford University Press, 2008; 64–6

Q3 Arterial Line

a) **Why is invasive blood pressure monitoring used in ICU? (3 marks)**
b) **List complications that may occur following arterial cannulation (8 marks)**
c) **Describe the information that may be obtained from an arterial pressure waveform (9 marks)**

Aims

The ability to insert an arterial line is a core skill for anaesthetists, but we must be able to interpret what we see on the screen to guide clinical treatment.

a) Indications

- To provide beat-to-beat blood pressure monitoring, allowing instant evaluation of the cardiovascular response to clinical deterioration, inotropic or vasopressor treatment, or sedation administration
- Where non-invasive blood pressure may be inaccurate or unreliable (e.g. in the presence of arrhythmias, obesity)
- Serial arterial blood gas measurement or routine FBC, U&E, and clotting analysis
- Necessary for some types of cardiac output monitoring used in ICU e.g. LidCO, PICCO

b) Complications

- Bleeding: can be significant (e.g. femoral puncture and retroperitoneal collection)
- Haematoma following arterial puncture
- Distal ischaemia, leading to necrosis; especially following accidental drug injection
- Infection
- Retrograde embolic phenomenon
- Pseudo-aneurysm
- Arteriovenous fistula
- Compartment syndrome
- Damage to adjacent structures (i.e. tendon, nerve)
- Exsanguination following accidental disconnection
- Stenosis of vessel lumen

c) Information from Waveform

- Heart rate
- Peak systolic pressure
- Diastolic pressure
- Systolic pressure variation, or arterial trace 'swing' in mechanically ventilated patients. An exaggerated variation is associated with hypovolaemia
- Hypovolaemia may also be indicated by a low position of the dicrotic notch
- Stroke volume: the area under the systolic part of the arterial waveform forms the basis of pulse contour analysis cardiac output measuring devices
- Mean arterial pressure: often preferable as an endpoint for titrating inotrope or vasopressor therapy to support the circulation
- The slope of the upstroke reflects myocardial contractility; the systolic time interval or rate of pressure change per unit time (dP/dT) is inversely proportional to contractility
- The slope of the downstroke, i.e. diastolic decay, gives an idea of systemic vascular resistance: a slow fall indicates vasoconstriction and a sharp fall indicates vasodilatation

- Certain valve disease states may be suggested (e.g. a wide pulse pressure in aortic regurgitation, a slowed upstroke in aortic stenosis)

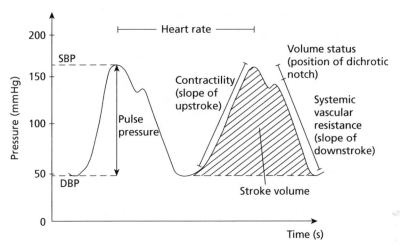

Figure 23. Arterial line trace

Notes

Reference

Ashley E. Arterial pressure monitoring. In: Waldmann C, Soni N, Rhodes A, eds. *Oxford Desk Reference: Critical Care*. Oxford University Press, 2008; 102–3

Q4 Cardiopulmonary Exercise Testing

a) **Describe how cardiopulmonary exercise testing (CPET) is performed and list the variables measured and derived (7 marks)**

b) **Define anaerobic threshold (AT) and outline its clinical relevance (6 marks)**

c) **List indications for use of CPET in surgical and non-surgical patients (7 marks)**

Aims

CPET is gaining popularity in the UK as a non-invasive investigation prior to major surgery. A basic understanding of the results is required in order to help clinicians to stratify risk and plan patients' perioperative care.

a) CPET

- The CPET set-up includes a bicycle ergonometer or treadmill, a 12-lead exercise ECG, a BP cuff, and a mouthpiece for the gas analyser, all connected to the test computer
- The subject pedals or runs for a determined period of time against an incremental resistance whilst respiratory, cardiovascular, and metabolic variables are collected and analysed

i) Variables measured
- FiO_2, EtO_2, VO_2 (O_2 consumption)
- $EtCO_2$, VCO_2 (CO_2 output)
- Tidal volume, respiratory rate, SpO_2, and work rate
- Heart rate, ST segment depression (ischaemia), non-invasive blood pressure

ii) Variables calculated
- Anaerobic threshold (AT)
- V_e/VCO_2 (minute ventilation per unit decrease of CO_2 production)

b) Definitions

- Anaerobic threshold (AT) is the O_2 consumption (mL/mg/min) at which the subject supplements aerobic metabolism with anaerobic metabolism in order to maintain appropriate VO_2 (the 'transition' point)
- At AT, VCO_2 ↑ disproportionately to VO_2, as excess lactic acid released from muscles is excreted via ↑ ventilation from the lungs, due to HCO_3 buffering
- AT can be calculated by the V-slope method (plotting VCO_2 against VO_2 and identifying the take-off from a line of unity). If AT occurs at a lower VO_2 level (<11mL/kg/min), particularly in association with ST segment changes, risk of surgical mortality is increased
- V_e/VCO_2 is the ratio of minute ventilation to volume of CO_2 produced and is a measure of the lung's ability to excrete CO_2. It is raised in severe COPD, heart failure, and pulmonary hypertension, and is used as an additional indicator of increased risk for major surgery

c) Indications for CPET

i) Surgical
- Indication of surgical morbidity and mortality for major thoracic, vascular, and abdominal surgery, including risk of postoperative cardiorespiratory complications
- Useful predictor for postoperative destination (i.e. ICU, HDU, or ward)

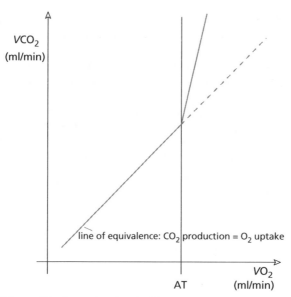

Figure 24. Anaerobic threshold

ii) Non-surgical
- Assessment of unexplained shortness of breath
- Prognosis in heart failure or post heart transplant
- Assessment of respiratory function in COPD or post lobectomy/pneumonectomy patients
- To assess the response to treatment for cystic fibrosis and pulmonary hypertension
- Functional assessment of recovery of survivors of multi-organ failure post ICU admission
- Assessment of fitness of athletes

Notes

References

Older P, Hall V. Preoperative evaluation of cardiac risk. *British Journal of Hospital Medicine (London)*, **66**: 452–7, 2005

Snowden CP, Prentis JM, Anderson HL, *et al.* Submaximal cardiopulmonary exercise testing predicts complications and hospital length of stay in patients undergoing major elective surgery. *Annals of Surgery*, **251**: 535–41, 2010

Wilson RJ, Davies S., Yates D, Redman J, Stone M. Impaired functional capacity is associated with all-cause mortality after major elective intra-abdominal surgery. *British Journal of Anaesthesia*, **105**: 297–303, 2010

Q5 Critical Care Analgesia

a) **List the causes of pain in ICU patients (4 marks)**

b) **Outline the adverse effects caused by pain in ICU patients (6 marks)**

c) **What methods of analgesia are available for pain relief in ICU? (10 marks)**

Aims

Pain is both difficult to assess and challenging to treat effectively in ICU. Candidates must be aware of the multi-modal therapies available.

a) Causes of Pain

Changes during ICU stay from acute to chronic

- Surgical incisions, trauma
- Organ dysfunction (e.g. GI ischaemia, venous thromboembolic disease (PE, DVT), cardiac ischaemia)
- Pre-existing (e.g. vascular, neuropathic, arthritis, malignancy)
- Procedures (e.g. dressing changes, turning, cannula insertion, tracheal suction)
- Pressure sores, wounds, joint pains, contractures from prolonged immobility
- Chronic pain conditions (e.g. myopathy, neuropathy)

b) Adverse Effects of Pain

- Cardiovascular: increased sympathetic drive $\rightarrow$ $\uparrow$HR/BP $\rightarrow$ myocardial O_2 demand outstripping supply $\rightarrow$ ischaemia and infarction
- Respiratory: atelectasis, increased O_2 consumption, V/Q mismatch, impaired gas exchange
- Gastrointestinal: nausea and vomiting, ileus
- Genitourinary: urinary retention causing agitation
- Endocrine: $\uparrow$ stress response causes $\uparrow$ aldosterone and ADH secretion, $\uparrow$ Na^+ and H_2O retention
- Haematological: increased risk of venous stasis, and thus DVT and PE
- Musculoskeletal: immobility leads to development of critical illness polyneuropathy and myopathy; pain due to pressure from the pulse oximetry probe or BP cuff
- Neuropsychological: sleep deprivation, agitation, and delirium $\uparrow$ the chances of developing post-traumatic stress disorder
- $\uparrow$ length of stay in ICU

c) Methods of Analgesia

i) Paracetamol
- Simple analgesic and antipyretic
- IV infusion if PO, NG, PR unavailable
- Evidence that opiate requirements are reduced

ii) Opioids
- Morphine, alfentanil, and fentanyl infusions are the mainstay for an analgesic regimen. Practice is changing due to accumulation and slower metabolism in prolonged infusions
- Remifentanil: has properties of the ideal ICU opioid agent (short context-sensitive half-life)
  - Provides excellent analgo-sedation; often possible to use it as a sole sedative
  - Allows efficient neurological assessment when required

- Cardiovascularly stable and an excellent choice for patients with impaired renal and liver function
- Quicker time to extubation and discharge: potentially attractive pharmaco-economically

iii) Other agents
- Clonidine: α_2 agonist also used for treatment of delirium and hypertension. Side effects include cardiovascular depression, ↓ gut motility, and potentially ↑ blood glucose levels
- Ketamine: phencyclidine derivative used for excellent analgesic properties in procedures such as dressing change in burns patients. Also used for sedation and treatment of severe asthma or COPD exacerbation. Side effects include CVS stimulation, nausea and vomiting, ↑ secretions, and emergence delirium
- Neuropathic analgesics: neuropathic pain in ICU patients is difficult to treat with a standard regimen. Consider using drugs such as tricyclic antidepressants, gabapentin, and pregabalin. Ensure pre-admission regimen in patients with long-standing neuropathic pain is continued
- NSAIDs: good opioid-sparing effects but side-effect profile (e.g. renal, anti-platelet, GI ulceration) is often incompatible with critical care use

iv) Regional Anaesthesia
- Epidural: used primarily for postoperative analgesia or 'flail-chest' injuries. Superior analgesia provides quicker ventilator weaning and optimal respiratory function. Standard risks apply for epidural catheter insertion and local anaesthetic infusion (e.g. insertion in the presence of coagulopathy, anti-platelet agent therapy, or sepsis)
- Other: interpleural catheters (inserted for chest wall trauma, breast surgery); any other indwelling catheters for peripheral nerve blockade
- Alternative therapies (e.g. TENS, aromatherapy): no evidence to support use in ICU patients, but therapies should not be withheld. Anecdotal evidence exists showing a benefit from acupuncture in neuropathic pain, and decreased analgesic requirements post aromatherapy!

Notes

Reference

Waldmann C. Pain management in ICU. In: Waldmann C, Soni N, Rhodes A, eds. *Oxford Desk Reference: Critical Care*. Oxford University Press, 2008; 508–9

Q6 Fat Embolism

A 54-year-old woman develops hypoxia, tachypnoea, and a widespread rash over her upper body 48 hours post intermedullary nailing for a displaced tibial fracture.

a) List the differential diagnoses of this presentation (4 marks)

b) What other clinical features may be present in fat embolism syndrome? (8 marks)

c) How do clinicians reduce the risk of and treat fat embolism? (8 marks)

Aims

This topic has appeared recently in the SAQ examination and, as such, may be repeated. The last part of the question includes areas which are still under research—supportive therapy should be emphasized over the controversial areas.

a) Differential Diagnoses

- Fat embolism syndrome
- Respiratory: LRTI, PE, atelectasis, pulmonary oedema, ARDS, pleural effusion
- Cardiac: MI, cardiac failure, arrhythmias
- Other: e.g. drug allergy, pain

b) Fat Embolism Syndrome

- Commonly presents 24–72 hours post injury/insult
- i) Respiratory Symptoms
  - Range from dyspnoea, tachypnoea, and hypoxia to a respiratory-failure-like picture requiring intubation and mechanical ventilation
- ii) Petechial Rash
  - Upper trunk (including axilla and neck), buccal membranes, conjunctiva
- iii) Neurological Symptoms:
  - Range from confusion or drowsiness through to seizures and coma. Focal signs (e.g. cranial nerve palsies) may also be present
- iv) Less Common
  - CVS compromise: tachycardia, arrhythmias, clotting derangement (e.g. DIC), renal impairment, retinopathy (Purtscher retinopathy)

c) Prevention and Treatment

- Important factors: preventative measures, early diagnosis, and supportive treatment
- i) Surgical Prevention
  - Early fracture immobilization and splinting
  - Intramedullary nailing within 24 hours is proven to ↓ trauma complication rates, but must be balanced against the risk of inducing further embolism, intraoperative blood loss, and length of operation
  - For trauma patients with significant pulmonary injuries, temporary external fixation is the preferred technique, with a subsequent intramedullary nailing when the patient has stabilized
  - Care should be taken to limit intra-osseous pressures during surgery

ii) Non-surgical Prevention
   - Prophylactic steroid administration in high-risk groups remains controversial
   - Supportive: oxygenation, ventilation, hydration, cardiovascular stability, DVT prophylaxis, care bundles (e.g. nutrition and stress ulcer prophylaxis)
   - Treatment with steroids, aspirin, and heparin remains controversial

Notes

References

Gupta A, Reilly CS. Fat embolism. *Continuing Education in Anaesthesia, Critical Care & Pain*, **7**: 148–51, 2007

Pape HC, Giannoudis P, Krettek C. The timing of fracture treatment in polytrauma patients: relevance of damage control orthopedic surgery. *American Journal of Surgery*, **183**: 622–9, 2002

Q7 Influenza Pandemic

A 45-year-old woman has been admitted to ICU from a medical ward with worsening respiratory failure following a four-day history of influenza-like illness

a) What are the management principles of this patient on arrival to ICU? (13 marks)

b) List methods for reducing cross-infection including the use of personnel protective equipment (PPE) (7 marks)

Aims

The recent worldwide influenza pandemic has affected ICU management and bed planning. The management of a pregnant woman with H1N1 influenza featured recently in the SAQ section of the examination, again highlighting the popularity of topical issues.

a) Management

  i) Early
  - Treat as for community-acquired pneumonia and sepsis
  - Intubate and ventilate if progressive deterioration of cardiorespiratory function
  - Initiate the early resuscitation bundle for sepsis (oxygen, fluids, inotropes, vasopressors)
  - Commence invasive haemodynamic monitoring
  - Obtain multiple peripheral blood cultures and commence broad-spectrum antibiotics according to local guidelines if evidence of bacterial co-infection
  - Send throat and nasopharyngeal swabs or endotracheal aspirates for influenza testing
    - Rapid influenza diagnostic test (performed in 30 minutes, variable sensitivity to specific influenza strains)
    - Real-time reverse transcriptase-polymerase chain reaction test (results take 2–4 days, highly sensitive to specific strains)
    - Others: viral culture and direct immunofluorescence assay
  - If positive influenza results obtained, commence appropriate antivirals with microbiology advice
  - If not intubated, caution with NIV if influenza is suspected because of risk of cross-infection

  ii) Late
  - Ventilator care bundle including protective lung ventilation strategies
  - Continued microbiological input regarding appropriate antimicrobials if positive blood cultures
  - Thromboprophylaxis
  - Consider activated protein C if evidence of severe septic shock and criteria are fulfilled
  - Renal replacement therapy (if evidence of renal impairment)
  - Methods for improving oxygenation if respiratory function continues to deteriorate: proning, high-frequency oscillatory ventilation, consultation with regional ECMO centre
  - Limit corticosteroid use in critically ill influenza patients to treating confirmed adrenal suppression or bronchospasm/asthma; increases susceptibility to opportunistic infections

b) Methods

- Patient ideally nursed in single side-room with adequate ventilation (>12 air changes/hour)
- Limited visiting from relatives and friends; those who visit are instructed in hand hygiene

For Staff
- *If no close contact with patient:* hand hygiene and water-repellent mask
- *If close contact with patient (i.e. <3 feet away):* hand hygiene and gloves, plastic apron, mask
- *Aerosol-generated procedure (e.g. intubation, suctioning, bronchoscopy):*
  - hand hygiene and gloves, plastic apron, gown
  - filtering face piece 3 (FFP-3) respirator or mask (in UK)
  - eye protection with a visor or goggles

Notes

References

Patel M, Dennis A, Flutter C, Khan Z. Pandemic (H1N1) 2009 influenza. *British Journal of Anaesthesia*, **104**: 128–42, 2010

Rivers E, Nguyen B, Havstad S, *et al.* Early goal-directed therapy in the treatment of severe sepsis and septic shock. *New England Journal of Medicine*, **345**: 1368–77, 2001

UK Influenza Pandemic Contingency Plan. London: UK Health Departments, 2005

Q8 Guillain–Barré Syndrome

You have been asked to assess a 53-year-old woman on the medical ward who has developed motor weakness and breathing difficulties. You suspect she may have developed Guillain–Barré syndrome (GBS).

a) Outline clinical features to support your diagnosis (6 marks)

b) List specific investigations required to diagnose GBS (6 marks)

c) Describe the management of this syndrome (8 marks)

Aims

The pathogenesis and management of this syndrome are commonly examined because of its respiratory effects and requirement for critical care support. Although it is relatively rare, a core level of knowledge is required for optimal assessment and treatment.

a) Clinical Features

- Prodrome phase (*Campylobacter jejuni*, *Mycoplasma pneumoniae*, cytomegalovirus, Epstein–Barr virus (EBV), vaccines, major surgery)
- Progressive ascending symmetrical limb weakness
- Distal paraesthesia, pain, sensory loss
- Reduced or absent reflexes
- Nerve palsies (e.g. facial nerve, or rarely bulbar nerve)
- Respiratory muscle involvement; may ultimately require IPPV
- Autonomic dysfunction: tachycardia, arrhythmias, diaphoresis, urinary retention

b) Investigations

- Regular assessment of vital capacity (VC): transfer to HDU or ICU if VC <20mL/kg
- CSF analysis: ↑ protein and normal WCC
- Nerve conduction studies: to distinguish between axonal damage and demyelination
- MRI brain and spinal cord
- Blood tests
  - Antiganglioside autoantibodies
  - Antibodies and serology for: *C.jejuni, M.pneumoniae,* EBV, HSV, HIV, hepatitis A, B, C, atypical
  - TFTs, B_{12} and folate, paraprotein bands
- Stool and urine sample: *C.jejuni*, poliovirus, porphyrins

c) Management

- Transfer to HDU/ICU if evidence of respiratory compromise, bulbar involvement, or autonomic instability

i) Airway and Breathing
  - If VC<15mL/kg, intubate and ventilate
  - Suxamethonium is contraindicated (potential for fatal hyperkalaemia)
  - Consider early tracheostomy; potential for prolonged respiratory wean

ii) Circulation
  - Caution with CVS instability during anaesthesia for intubation because of autonomic dysfunction

- CVS support may be required: e.g. pacing for treatment-resistant severe bradyarrhythmias

iii) Drugs and Disability
  - IV immunoglobulins (IgG): 400mg/kg OD for 5 days
  - Plasma exchange: 400mL/kg, 3–5 treatments over 5–8 days
  - Early physiotherapy to prevent flexion contractures, pressure sores, nerve palsies
  - Psychiatric input (cognitive disturbances and depression are common)

iv) Other
  - Thromboprophylaxis
  - Early enteral feeding (or parenteral route if ileus present) and stress ulcer prophylaxis
  - Analgesia: consider neuropathic analgesics (e.g. gabapentin, amitriptyline)

Notes

Reference

Smith M, Pritchard C. Guillain-Barre syndrome. In: Waldmann C, Soni N, Rhodes A, eds. *Oxford Desk Reference: Critical Care*. Oxford University Press, 2008; 372–3

Q9 GIFTASUP

You are called to the ward to review a 69-year-old man 24 hours post laparoscopic right hemicolectomy. He has been vomiting and is now oliguric, passing 15mL of urine over the last 2 hours.

a) Describe your initial management (8 marks)

b) Discuss the pros and cons of using the following fluids for resuscitation in this patient (12 marks)

i) 0.9% saline

ii) Hartmann's solution

iii) 5% dextrose solution

iv) colloid (all forms)

Aims

Recently published guidelines (GIFTASUP) provide a rigid framework for any question to be built around, including perioperative fluid infusion. Knowledge of these documents allows the candidate to tackle broad topics in a structured manner and appear up to date with current opinion and literature.

a) Initial Management

- Structured approach to patient: assess airway, breathing, and circulation
- Assessment of filling status
  - fluid balance including during surgery
  - skin turgor
  - CVP
  - peripheral capillary refill time
  - HR and BP
- Information about preoperative renal function may help indicate renal reserve
- ABG: rapid assessment of metabolic and electrolyte status
- Assess fluid status
  - Hypovolaemia
    - Pre-renal failure secondary to fluid depletion
    - Assess and review response to fluid bolus of 200mL crystalloid
    - Continue until patient is euvolaemic and urine output has improved (>1ml/kg/hr)
  - Euvolaemia
    - Intrinsic acute kidney injury or post-renal obstruction to be considered
    - Stop potentially nephrotoxic drugs (e.g. aminoglycosides, NSAIDs)
    - Ultrasound scan to rule out post-renal obstruction (will also give information on size on kidneys, possible indicator of underlying chronic renal disease)
    - If patient remains anuric, assess perfusion pressure
    - If low, consider augmenting BP with vasopressors or inotropes in HDU/ICU
    - May need haemofiltration and renal team input

b) Fluid Resuscitation

- The GIFTASUP consensus guidelines establish scenarios which suggest that certain fluids may have advantages over others

i) 0.9% Saline

Advantages
- Crystalloid, therefore rehydrates all fluid spaces well
- Low incidence of anaphylaxis or allergy
- High sodium load in sodium-depleted patients (i.e. free-water clearance impaired, hyponatraemic) Chloride load for replacement of gastric fluid, i.e. in excessive vomiting

Disadvantages
- Excessive infusion of chloride associated with metabolic acidosis
- Risk of hypernatraemia in patients with impaired sodium clearance
- Low pH makes the term 'normal saline' a fallacy

ii) Hartmann's Solution

Advantages
- As for 0.9% saline
- Less acidotic than 0.9% saline
- Balanced salt solution for better rehydration of intracellular and extracellular space
- ↓ electrolyte disturbance compared with other crystalloid solutions
- ↓ Na^+ and Cl^- load for patients with impaired Na^+ clearance postoperatively due to acute phase response

Disadvantages
- Lactate can accumulate in patients with liver failure
- May contribute to hyperglycaemia in diabetic patients
- Caution in patients with acute kidney injury as K^+ accumulation possible, although evidence base justifies its use and safety profile

iii) Dextrose

Advantages
- Acts as a source of free water in water-depleted patients (i.e. hypernatraemia)
- Distributed to all body compartments, with expansion of intracellular compartment more than other crystalloids

Disadvantages
- Poor for intravascular volume expansion
- Associated with deranged cellular function, oedema, deranged blood sugar in diabetics; can precipitate hyponatraemia and fluid overload

iv) Colloid

Advantages
- Theoretical advantage of plasma expansion longer than crystalloids to maintain circulation and perfusion
- Reduces oedema risk as smaller equivalent volume of fluid should be required to restore BP

Disadvantages
- Poor for hypovolaemia because of fluid depletion
- Risk of allergic or anaphylactic response
- Large molecule starches associated with increase in acute kidney injury in oliguric patients
- Duration of plasma expansion often short lived

References

Powell-Tuck J, Gosling P, Lobo, DN, *et al. British Consensus Guidelines on Intravenous Fluid Therapy for Adult Surgical Patients (GIFTASUP)*, 2009
http://www.bapen.org.uk/pdfs/bapen_pubs/giftasup.pdf (accessed 1 December 2010)

Q10 Hypothermia

A 68-year-old man has been successfully resuscitated following an out-of-hospital VF cardiac arrest.

a) Describe the initial management of this patient in the Emergency Department upon return of spontaneous cardiac output (ROSC) (9 marks)

b) Discuss the principles and complications of elective hypothermia in ICU treatment post VF arrest (11 marks)

Aims

Areas of this SAQ are still controversial, but awareness of this topic is important for both examination purposes and the ongoing treatment of survivors of cardiac arrest

a) Management Aims

- Assess the adequacy of the CVS
- Identify the trigger for the original pathological rhythm
- Grade the degree of damage to organ systems sustained during arrest
- Basic observations:
  - HR and rhythm, 12-lead ECG
  - blood pressure
  - oxygen saturations
  - temperature
  - ABG
  - chest radiograph
  - blood sugar if not obtained during resuscitation phase
  - FBC, U&E, troponin, clotting, and cross-match
- Collateral history from next of kin, GP, patient's notes; paramedics to identify VF precipitant
- Depending on precipitating factor, the patient may be transferred for further interventional procedures (e.g. percutaneous angiography or intra-aortic balloon pump insertion)
- Transfer to ICU for further investigations, support, monitoring, and stabilization
- Referral to cardiology or the general medical registrar on call for further investigations (e.g. echocardiography)

b) Elective Hypothermia

- Elective hypothermia has been shown to improve neurological recovery in patients successfully resuscitated from VF out-of-hospital cardiac arrests
- Two large multicentred RCTs in Australia and Europe found significant improvement in cognitive function in this cohort on discharge and at 6 months
- The principle is based on reducing cerebral metabolic oxygen consumption by reducing total entropy within the CNS
  - A 1°C ↓ in temperature correlates with a 6–8 % ↓ in metabolic rate and a change in CSF expression of neurochemical markers
  - Poor cerebral blood flow can persist for several hours following ROSC, and this is the basis for continuing for 24 hours
- Both studies aimed for a core temperature of 33–34°C for 24 hours post initial event
- However, both studies were small and the time taken to achieve core temperatures within range was long, averaging 8 hours

- The difference in outcome was significant only in VF or VT arrests following baseline adjustments of the data
- Complications associated with cooling
  - Electrolyte abnormalities, especially K^+ and Mg^{2+}
  - Trend towards an increase in sepsis in the European study, possibly representing impaired neutrophil function
  - Difficulty in predicting drug metabolism and clearance, especially important when assessing neurological recovery or when paralysing agents have been used to prevent shivering
- The International Liaison Committee on Resuscitation has integrated this into their most recent guidelines as best care for patients post VF arrest
- Current research is focused around techniques to improve the rate and maintenance of hypothermia, the duration of cooling, and other cohorts who may benefit.

Notes

References

Bernard SA, Buist MD. Induced hypothermia in the intensive care unit: a review. *Critical Care Medicine*, **31**: 2041–51, 2003

Bernard SA, Gray TW, Buist MD, *et al*. Treatment of comatose survivors of out-of-hospital cardiac arrest with induced hypothermia. *New England Journal of Medicine*, **346**: 557–63, 2002

Zeiner A, Holzer M, Sterz F, *et al*. Mild resuscitative hypothermia to improve neurological outcome after cardiac arrest. A clinical feasibility trial. Hypothermia After Cardiac Arrest (HACA) Study Group. *Stroke*, **31**: 86–94, 2000

Q11 ICU Admission and Discharge

a) **Outline the potential criteria for patient admission to ICU (10 marks)**

b) **How is it decided when a patient should be discharged from ICU and what factors should be taken into account to ensure that discharge is successful? (10 marks)**

Aims

Assessing acutely unwell patients for suitability for ICU admission is a common task for critical care physicians, especially at the grade likely to be sitting the final FRCA. It is difficult to provide a structured approach covering all aspects of both patients and their pathology. The same is also true for discharging patients from the unit.

a) Criteria for ICU Admission

- Patients may be admitted to a critical care area from the operating theatre, the recovery area, the Emergency Department, or hospital wards
- Patients admitted from wards to ICU have ↑ percentage mortality than those admitted from elsewhere; a longer hospital stay prior to ICU admission also increases mortality
- Because of lack of beds, difficult decisions are made in allocating limited ICU resources; however, timely admission without delay may be crucial if patients are to benefit
- Patients may be refused admission because of lack of beds or because they are thought to be too sick to benefit so that admission would be futile
- Others are denied access because it is felt that they are not sick enough and that care available on a ward is satisfactory.
- All admissions and refused admissions should be discussed with the ICU consultant and a management plan drawn up
- The ICU consultant should see all admissions within 12 hours or less if appropriate
- Unfortunately, coping with death at home or on the wards has become more challenging, and patients with a small chance of recovery are admitted to ICU essentially as that is where death is better managed
- A national audit of medical patients admitted to ICU who subsequently died found that many had profound physiological abnormalities for hours before ICU admission with considerable shortcomings in their management whilst on the ward
- This has been the catalyst for developing outreach and medical emergency teams; although evidence for their effectiveness has not been confirmed by trials (e.g. MERIT)
- More recently, NICE has published a document (*The Acutely Ill Patient*) which has increased the profile of this group of sick patients on the wards

b) Ensuring a Successful Discharge

- A patient should be discharged from ICU when the condition leading to his/her admission has been resolved and adequately treated, and when the intensive care consultant considers that the patient would no longer benefit from available treatment
- There may be a wide variation in criteria for discharge, and this may depend upon institutional factors as well as the status of the patient
- About 30% of deaths in ICU patients occur after they are discharged from the ICU. The process of discharge and care received afterwards should not be ignored when attempting to minimize intensive care mortality

- Patients discharged prematurely have ↑ mortality and readmission rate; delaying discharge may be extremely important, especially at night. Ideally, discharge between 22:00 and 07:00 should be avoided and documented as an adverse incident
- ICU teams should discuss patients' problems directly with the ward team when they are discharged; extensive documentation is essential
- Readmissions to ICU have significantly ↑ mortality and length of stay. Planned discharges must take place when the patient no longer requires ICU support
- Outreach services often have responsibility for following up discharged patients; they provide a valuable link between ICU and the wards by sharing critical care skills and supporting patients and ward staff.
- Outreach in this form may ↓ ICU readmission rates and improve survival to discharge
- Patients (and their relatives) may have profound long-term psychological and physical sequelae from their ICU stay:
  - Rehabilitation programmes are beneficial
  - ICU follow-up clinics are now established and are extremely valuable in supporting these patients.
  - NICE has published guidelines for rehabilitation after ICU to ensure successful discharge and long-term improvement
  - Rehabilitation needs should be assessed and commenced when the patient is still in ICU, continued on the ward afterwards, and then continued once the patient is returned to the community

Notes

References

Goldfrad C, Rowan K. Consequences of discharges from intensive care at night. *Lancet*, **355**: 1138–42, 2000

Goldhill D, Waldmann C. Excellent anaesthesia needs patient preparation and postoperative support to influence outcome. *Current Opinion in Anaesthesiology*, **19**: 192–7, 2006

National Health Service Executive (NHSE). *Guidelines on Admission to and Discharge from Intensive Care and High Dependency Units*. London: Department of Health, 1996

NICE. *Rehabilitation Guidelines*. London: NICE, 2009

Q12 **ICU Anaemia**

a) **List the causes of anaemia in critically unwell patients (9 marks)**

b) **Outline potential risks associated with transfusion of packed red cells (11 marks)**

Aims

Transfusing blood can have significant clinical and financial implications, and appropriate decisions should be made, especially in ICU, as to the value of this action

a) Causes of Anaemia

i) Pre-existing disease state
- Iron, vitamin B_{12}, and folate deficiency
- Anaemia of chronic disease (e.g. renal failure)
- Haemoglobinopathies (e.g. sickle cell, thalassaemia)
- Chronic alcohol abuse
- Drugs: folate antagonists (e.g. phenytoin)
- Haematological (e.g. myelodysplastic syndrome)

ii) Acquired
- Loss of red blood cells
  - Surgical bleeding
  - Trauma
  - GI bleed
  - Destruction (i.e. haemofiltration, haemolytic disease)
  - Regular sampling
- Failure in haemopoesis
  - Multifactorial, behaves similarly to anaemia of chronic disease
  - ↓ production of erythropoietin (EPO)
  - ↓ sensitivity of red marrow to EPO
  - ↑ hepcidin production reduces serum iron availability

b) Risks of Transfusion

i) Immune
- Acute
  - Haemolysis due to ABO incompatibility
  - Anaphylaxis
  - Pyrexia
  - Transfusion-related acute lung injury
- Delayed
  - Haemolysis (7–10 days later)
  - Blood component reaction, i.e. plasma proteins, platelets (reducing following leucodepletion of red cells)
- Late
  - Rhesus exposure of Rh-negative women

ii) Infective (mainly viral)
- Hepatitis B and C screened for currently in UK
- HIV
- CJD: recipients of packed cells since 1980 are excluded from donating red blood cells
- Other (e.g. cytomegalovirus, malaria, syphilis, bacteria)

iii) Other
- Metabolic
  - Hyperkalaemia
  - Citrate toxicity (hypocalcaemia and metabolic alkalosis from citrate metabolism to yield bicarbonate)
- Hypothermia: stored red cells at 4°C
- Impaired O_2 delivery immediately post-transfusion due to ↓ 2,3-DPG and left shift of the O_2 dissociation curve
- Microparticulate emboli can form in stored blood
- Circulatory overload, especially during rapid administration
- Coagulopathy if transfusion limited to packed red cells

iv) Mortality
- The TRICC study showed a lower mortality in younger and healthier groups of ITU patients maintained at lower transfusion trigger compared with a liberal group
- Liberal transfusion also associated with more cardiac complications
- The CRIT study identified packed red cell transfusion during ITU stay as an independent predictor of mortality
- However, the SOAP study showed no association between mortality and transfusion requirements, possibly displaying the effects of leucodepletion introduction

Notes

....
....
....
....
....
....
....
....
....
....

References

Corwin HL, A. Gettinger, Pearl RG, et al. The CRIT study: anemia and blood transfusion in the critically ill—current clinical practice in the United States. *Critical Care Medicine*, **32**: 39–52, 2004

Hebert PC. Transfusion requirements in critical care (TRICC): a multicentre, randomized, controlled clinical study. Transfusion Requirements in Critical Care Investigators and the Canadian Critical care Trials Group. *British Journal of Anaesthesia*, **81 (Suppl 1)**: 25–33, 1998

http://www.shotuk.org/home/ (accessed 9 September 2009)

Vincent, J. L., Y. Sakr, et al. (2006). "Sepsis in European intensive care units: results of the SOAP study." *Crit Care Med* **34**(2): 344–353

Q13 **ICU Delirium**

a) **Define delirium (5 marks)**

b) **What are the consequences of delirium in the ICU? (4 marks)**

c) **Discuss how delirium may be assessed and detected in ICU (7 marks)**

d) **Outline the principles of delirium management (4 marks)**

Aims

All trainees have experienced the challenges of dealing with a confused ICU patient (usually at night!). Choosing the most appropriate course of action can have a profound influence on the clinical progress of the patient.

a) Definition

- A condition characterized by an acute change in mental status with a fluctuating course, characterized by inattention and disorganized thinking
- It is acute cerebral insufficiency and should be considered as an organ failure
- Occurs in 15–80% in critical care patients
- Three subtypes
  - Hyperactive: display agitation, restlessness, and emotional lability (10% of cases)
  - Hypoactive/hypokinetic: display decreased responsiveness, withdrawal, and apathy (often misdiagnosed as depression)
  - Mixed (45% of cases)

b) Consequences

- ↑ time on a ventilator and in intensive care
- ↑ incidence of unplanned extubation
- ↑ incidence of failed extubation
- Removal of lines and catheters
- 3× ↑ mortality
- ↑ cognitive decline long term

c) Assessment and Detection

- Adequate assessment of delirium requires optimal sedation of the patient
  - Ensure pain is adequately managed and the patient is minimally sedated
  - Include daily sedation holds
  - Analgosedation (e.g. remifentanil: only licensed for ICU use for 72 hours)
- There are a variety of sedation scores (e.g. Ramsay or Richmond Agitation–Sedation Scale (RASS) scores). With RASS the patient needs to be sedated at level 0 or –1 in order to assess delirium
- A screening tool for delirium should reliably evaluate the primary components of delirium:
  - consciousness
  - inattention
  - disorganized thinking
  - fluctuating course
  - be valid in a diverse critical care population
  - be completed quickly and easily
  - not require extra equipment or the presence of psychiatrist
- The tool commonly used is the Confusion Assessment Method in the ICU (CAM-ICU)

- This tool includes asking the patient to squeeze fingers when the letter 'A' is mentioned in 'SAVE A HAART'
- If this is done correctly, they are then tested on four simple questions (e.g. 'A stone floats on water. True or False?')
- Patients are CAM-ICU +ve or −ve. The assessment should be carried out at each change of nursing shift

d) Management

- Adequate pain control
- Ensure sepsis is controlled and sources of infection managed
- Ensure patient is not hypoxic and that there is biochemical stability
- Eliminate predisposing drugs such as benzodiazepines
- Pharmacological management
  - First line is incremental doses of haloperidol (monitor Q–Tc interval)
  - Olanzepine where haloperidol is not suitable
  - Consider trazadone at night

Notes

References

Ely EW, Inouye SK, Bernard GR, *et al.* Delirium in mechanically ventilated patients: validity and reliability of the confusion assessment method for the intensive care unit (CAM-ICU). *JAMA*, **286**: 2703–10, 2001

Pun BT, Gordon SM, Peterson JF, *et al.* Large-scale implementation of sedation and delirium monitoring in the intensive care unit: a report from two medical centers. *Critical Care Medicine* **33**: 1199–1205, 2005

Sessler CN, Gosnell MS, Grap MJ, *et al.* The Richmond Agitation–Sedation Scale: validity and reliability in adult intensive care unit patients. *American Journal of Respiratory and Critical Care Medicine*, **166**: 1338–44, 2002

http://www. icudelirium.co.uk (accessed 27 April 2010)

Q14 **ICU Rehabilitation**

a) **List common physical problems experienced by patients post critical illness (7 marks)**

b) **What other issues commonly occur following critical illness? (6 marks)**

c) **Outline the important principles in providing critical illness rehabilitation (7 marks)**

Aims

A large amount of interest is developing in patient outcome following discharge from critical care areas, and this question aims to explore your understanding of this emerging area of extended ICU practice.

a) Physical Problems

- Painful joints
- Muscle wasting
- Weakness
- Poor mobility
- Skin, hair, and nail disorders
- Taste loss and poor appetite
- Occasionally persistent renal dysfunction; post renal failure usually manifests as a low GFR
- Tracheostomy scarring and, rarely, tracheal stenosis
- Dyshabilitation
- Tiredness and chronic-fatigue-like syndrome
- Ongoing respiratory problems: post-ARDS PFT may be 80% of normal after 6 months
- Sexual dysfunction
- Chronic pain and possibly drug dependence
- Wound healing requiring input from stoma nurse and wound therapist for healing laparostomy
- Persistence of MRSA status and the stigma associated with this long term

b) Other Issues

- Anxiety and depression
- Post-traumatic stress disorder (PTSD) including features such as recurring nightmares, social withdrawal, marriage/relationship difficulties, and poor sleep patterns
- Long-term cognitive impairment including dysfunction of memory, attention and concentration, linguistic and numerical skills, and executive function
- Psychosexual dysfunction
- Financial problems
- Difficulties in returning to employment

c) Guidelines for Rehabilitation:

The recommendations of the NICE guidelines on critical illness rehabilitation (March 2009) cover the following areas:

i) Key Principles of Care
- Ensure continuity of care by coordinating the patient's rehabilitation care pathway
- Regular review and updating of short-term and medium-term goals

- Communication with primary and other healthcare settings for functional reassessment
- Ensure patient has access to self-directed rehabilitation manual

ii) During the Critical Care Stay
- Full clinical assessment to determine rehabilitation goals and needs, to commence rehabilitation as soon as possible, and to avoid of further morbidities

iii) Before Discharge from Critical Care
- Full clinical re-assessment of above points, identifying potential physical and psychological problems and updating rehabilitation goals

iv) During Ward-Based Care
- Further clinical re-assessment via a multidisciplinary team to form a structured personalized rehabilitation programme
- Identify psychological issues (e.g. PTSD) and refer to appropriate specialties

v) Before Discharge Home or to Community Care
- Functional assessment of physical and non-physical status, i.e. can the patient achieve their ADLs?
- Further update rehabilitation goals and ensure referral network is in place

vi) 2–3 Months after Discharge from Critical Care
- Review and re-assessment of functional status as above
- Assessment of progress: are they achieving rehabilitation goals?
- Further referrals for psychological counselling if appropriate

Notes

References

Schweickert WD, Pohlman MC, Pohlman AS, *et al.* (2009). Early physical and occupational therapy in mechanically ventilated, critically ill patients: a randomised controlled trial. *Lancet*, **373**: 1874–82
http://guidance.nice.org.uk/CG83 (accessed 4 October 2009)

Q15 ICU Sedation

a) Why is sedation important in intensive care? (8 marks)

b) What is sedation scoring? (7 marks)

c) Define 'optimal sedation' (5 marks)

Aims

The skill and challenge of providing optimal sedation for ICU patients, similarly to treating delirium, can have a marked effect on their clinical progress.

a) Importance of Sedation

- Most ICU patients require some form of sedation to make them comfortable during their ICU stay
- In some countries concern about the use of sedative drugs has led to the use of restraint, but the recent pan-European initiative PRICE (Patient Restraint in Intensive Care patients) has demonstrated that restraint on its own is not a good thing
- Under-sedation: patient discomfort, increased risk of loss of airway and vascular access, and therefore poor outcome
- Over-sedation: hypotension, undetected delirium, prolonged ventilatory and intensive care time, ileus, immobility, and critical illness neuropathy and myopathy
- Long-term: post-traumatic stress disorder (PTSD)
- Therefore a balanced approach to sedation is necessary
- Daily sedation interruption reduces time on the ventilator; this has become common practice
- Propofol, particularly in children, was associated with fatal metabolic acidosis when used in excess

b) Sedation Scoring

- Assessment of depth of patient sedation to meet patient-specific objectives:
  - patient comfort
  - pain control
  - reduction of anxiety
  - facilitation of nursing care
  - sleep management
  - avoidance of adverse outcomes (e.g. PTSD)
- No consensus in international guidelines regarding which scale to use
- Assessment methods have generally been compared with each other
- Validation is problematic; lack of an objective standard to validate against
- How to choose a scale?
  - Ease of use
  - Familiarity
  - Ability to be used in a consistent and standardized way
  - Usability in tandem with other scoring systems (e.g. for pain and delirium)
- Two commonly used scales are the Ramsay score and the Richmond Agitation–Sedation Score

c) Optimal Sedation

- Refers to use of best-evidence methods for sedating the patient appropriately so that he/she is neither over-sedated nor under-sedated
- There are several aspects
  - Use of analgosedation rather than hypnotic-based sedation
  - Use of sedation holding
  - Reduce the need for imaging for slow-waking
  - Reduce time spent on the ventilator and on ICU
  - Enable rehabilitation from day 1 to help prevent post-ICU weakness
  - Reduce incidence of post-ICU psychological problems (e.g. PTSD)
  - Sedation scoring to ensure patient is awake enough (except with severe ARDS) to be assessed for delirium

Notes

References

De Jonghe B, Cook D, Appere-de-Vecchi C, Guyatt G, Meade M, Outin H Using and understanding sedation scoring systems: a systematic review. *Intensive Care Medicine*, **26**: 275–85, 2000

Jacobi J, Fraser GL, Coursin DB, *et al*. Clinical practice guidelines for the sustained use of sedatives and analgesics in the critically ill adult. *Critical Care Medicine*, **30**: 119–41, 2002

Reschreiter H, Maiden M, Kapila A. Sedation practice in the intensive care unit: a UK national survey. *Critical Care*, **12**: R152, 2008

Sessler CN, Gosnell MS, Grap MJ, *et al*. The Richmond Agitation–Sedation Scale: validity and reliability in adult intensive care unit patients. *American Journal of Respiratory and Critical Care Medicine*, **166**: 1338–44, 2002

Q16 ICU Weakness

a) List potential causes of weakness in a critically unwell patient (10 marks)

b) Define critical illness myopathy (CIM) and critical illness polyneuropathy (CIP) (4 marks)

c) What investigations help to distinguish between CIM and CIP? (6 marks)

Aims

This type of question is best answered in a structured manner. The system we have used is anatomically based, working from the CNS where the impulses are generated out to the peripheral muscles where the response to stimulus is elicited.

a) Causes of Weakness

i) CNS
   - Coma or ↓ GCS: therefore not generating impulses required for purposeful movement; may be due to disease process or deep sedation
   - Central primary pathology causing CNS injury (e.g. stroke or intracranial bleed)
   - Exacerbation of pre-existing CNS disease, i.e. Parkinson's disease or multiple sclerosis
   - Non-convulsive status or post-ictal patients
   - Guillain-Barré disease: difficult to classify as affects both CNS and PNS
   - Alcohol abuse and vitamin deficiencies (often related)

ii) Spinal Cord
   - Trauma 2° to disruption or ischaemia
   - Myelitis
   - Spinal cord infarction
   - Infection (usually viral): previously polio, now West Nile virus

iii) CNS–PNS junction
   - Epidural mass effect secondary to abscess or haematoma compressing nerves leaving ventral horn

iv) PNS
   - Trauma disrupting the continuity of axon trunks
   - Compression-induced degeneration, i.e. patient positioning or haematoma following trauma or intravascular line
   - Peripheral demyelination
   - Guillain-Barré disease (as above)
   - Alcohol and vitamin deficiencies (as above)

v) Neuromuscular Junction
   - Receptor deficiency (e.g. myasthenia gravis)
   - Accumulation of NDMB in patients with ↓ hepatic or renal clearance
   - Acquired or genetic deficiency of pseudo-cholinesterase post suxamethonium administration
   - Hypokalaemia, hypermagnesaemia, hypophosphotaemia
   - Hypothermia

vi) Musculoskeletal
   - Critical illness myopathy—four histological subclasses exist:
     - necrotising (worst muscle recovery)
     - cachectic

- ◆ acute rhabdomyolysis
- ◆ thick filament (myosin) loss
- Fracture, dislocation
- Compartment syndrome with resultant neuromuscular ischaemia

vii) Other drugs
- Steroids, aminoglycosides

b) CIM and CIP

If CIM and CIP occur together, this is termed critical illness neuromyopathy

i) Critical Illness Myopathy
- Acute-onset muscular weakness due to muscle inflammation and death with normal nerve conduction patterns, usually occurring after the first week in ICU
- The muscle cannot be stimulated, even using direct stimulation
- Affects distal limbs, often associated with wasting
- Can also affect respiratory (intercostals and diaphragm) and ocular muscles

ii) Critical Illness Polyneuropathy
- Acute-onset polyneuropathy with normal muscle architecture and action
- Axonal degeneration, predominantly motor but can affect sensory axons
- Areflexia ± sensory deficit may be present
- Similar distribution to CIM but onset within 2–5 days

c) Investigations

i) Electrophysiological
- Nerve conduction studies
  - ◆ CIM: normal
  - ◆ CIP: ↓ compound muscle action potential (CMAP) and sensory action potential + normal conduction velocity
- EMG: abnormal with CIM during conscious cooperative movements

ii) Direct Muscle Stimulation
- Differentiates CIP from CIM in unconscious patients
  - ◆ CIP: ↓ or absent CMAP following nerve stimulation, but direct muscle stimulation produces normal contraction
  - ◆ CIM: CMAP ↓ or absent with both motor nerve stimulation and direct muscle stimulation

iii) Muscle Biopsy
- Invasive and slow to yield results
- Allows sub-classification of CIM and excludes other diagnoses, i.e. demyelination

iv) Serum Creatine Kinase
- Variably raised, but normal level does not exclude the diagnosis
- Massively elevated levels may suggest alternative pathology, i.e. rhabdomyolysis

Notes

Q17 **Non-invasive Ventilation**

a) **List i) the indications (7 marks) and ii) the contraindications (5 marks) for using non-invasive ventilation (NIV)**

b) **What are the benefits of using NIV? (5 marks)**

c) **Outline complications that may arise from NIV (3 marks)**

Aims

As a common source of referrals for critical care input, the appropriate and inappropriate use of non-invasive ventilation links to multiple areas, including who should or should not be suitable, where is the safest place for it to be performed, and the underlying physiological principles behind its use.

a) NIV

i) Indications
- Treatment of hypoxaemic respiratory failure (type 1 respiratory failure)
  - Conditions such as pneumonia, immunocompromise, post-pneumonectomy
- Treatment of acute hypercapnic respiratory failure (type 2 respiratory failure)
  - Commonly secondary to acute exacerbation of COPD
  - Indicated in mild to moderate acidosis (pH <7.3 and >7.25)
- To aid weaning of invasive ventilation (e.g. COPD)
- Post-extubation or tracheostomy decannulation failure: ↓ re-intubation rates with early introduction in high-risk patients
- Cardiogenic pulmonary oedema
- Useful in patients where intubation is contraindicated (e.g. patient refusal, palliation)
- Asthma: some evidence that benefit exists
- Neuromuscular disease (e.g. in Guillain–Barré syndrome, muscular dystrophy)

ii) Contraindications
- Need for immediate intubation due to worsening organ dysfunction: either worsening respiratory function or non-respiratory organ failure (e.g. haemodynamic instability, GI bleed, severe encephalopathy)
- Cardiorespiratory arrest
- Facial or upper airway trauma
- Loss of airway patency (e.g. GCS <8)
- Excessive airway secretions
- Lack of cooperation with high aspiration risk

b) Benefits of NIV

- Improves alveolar ventilation and ↓ work of breathing
- ↓ in morbidity and mortality, intubation rates, and treatment failure rates
- Cost-effective: ↓ length of hospital stay, avoidance of ICU stay and tracheostomy
- Avoids side effects of tracheal intubation (e.g. trauma to mucosa and teeth, tracheal stenosis, altered haemodynamics due to induction agents or pressor response)
- Patients can be managed on dedicated wards or intermediate areas
- Avoids need for sedation (and additional physiological side-effects) to tolerate a tracheal tube

c) Complications

- Local skin damage secondary to apparatus (e.g. bridge of nose, forehead, scalp)
- Gastric dilatation
- Ocular irritation and sinus congestion
- Difficulties in compliance because of discomfort and inability to communicate, eat, and drink
- May worsen secretion clearance, thus, increasing risk of infection/worsening respiratory failure

Notes

Reference

Singh S. Non-invasive positive pressure ventilation (NIPPV). In: Waldmann C, Soni N, Rhodes A, eds. *Oxford Desk Reference: Critical Care.* Oxford University Press, 2008; 30–1

Q18 Outreach

a) What levels of care exist with reference to patients' critical care needs? (5 marks)

b) Outline the role of the critical care outreach team? (6 marks)

c) Discuss important factors which guide hospitals in the care of the acutely ill patient (9 marks)

Aims

Modification of out-of-hours working has created multidisciplinary teams to manage patients and this extends to critical care. The outreach team forms a valuable part of the ICU team in both assessing and managing admissions whilst also following up discharges. These roles have been outlined in recently published guidelines which make questions like this easier to answer.

a) Levels of Care

- Level 0: patients whose needs can be met through normal ward care in an acute hospital
- Level 1: patients at risk of condition deteriorating or those recently relocated from higher levels of care whose needs can be met on an acute ward with additional advice and support from the critical care team
- Level 2: patients requiring more detailed observation or intervention including support for a single failing organ system and postoperative care, and those stepping down from higher levels of care
- Level 3: patients requiring advanced respiratory support alone, or basic respiratory support and support of at least two organ systems. Includes all complex patients requiring support for multi-organ failure

b) Role of Outreach Team

- Outreach services need to be developed as an integral part of each NHS organization's critical care service
- Aim to provide a hospital-wide approach to critical illness in collaboration with other hospital departments
- Main Objectives
  - To avoid unnecessary admissions: early recognition of deteriorating patients and helping institute appropriate treatment
  - To facilitate early admission to critical care to prevent further morbidity and mortality
  - To enable critical care discharges back to the ward with continued support and follow-up
  - To share critical care skills and expertise with multidisciplinary staff on the ward and in the community
  - To promote continuity of care
  - To ensure that outreach audit processes and feedback are established to facilitate improved services in the future

c) Guidelines: Acutely Ill Patients in Hospitals

- NICE guidelines on acutely ill patients in hospital published in 2007
- Physiological observations must be recorded at admission or first assessment
- A clear plan should be made regarding frequency and type of observations according to comorbidities, diagnosis, and treatment plan

- All acute patients should be monitored using a 'track and trigger' scoring system, with the ability to increase and decrease the frequency of monitoring according to physiological status
- NHS organizations must ensure that all staff caring for acute patients have adequate and appropriate training, education, and assessment of performing observations, monitoring, and the recognition of clinically deteriorating patients
- Patients must be grouped into low, medium, and high by their risk of clinical deterioration, and a suitable response by staff assigned according to group status
- Critical care referral for patients should be on a consultant-to-consultant basis
- Discharge of a patient from critical care to the ward should ideally take place in daylight hours, i.e. between 07:00 and 22:00 if possible
- Once the decision has been made to discharge the patient from critical care, it is the joint responsibility of ward staff and critical care staff to ensure safe transfer, a formal structured handover to identify further management plans, and the ability of the ward to carry out the continuing treatment

Notes

References

Department of Health. *Comprehensive Critical Care. A Review of Adult Critical Care Services*. London: Department of Health, 2000; 14–15

Intensive Care Society. *Guidelines for the Introduction of Outreach Services*. London: Intensive Care Society, 2002

Intensive Care Society. *Levels of critical care for adult patients*. London: Intensive Care Society, 2002

National Institute for Clinical Excellence. *Acutely Ill Patients in Hospital*, 2007

http://guidance.nice.org.uk/CG64 (accessed 5th October 2009)

Q19 Pancreatitis

A 42-year-old man has been admitted to the ICU with severe acute pancreatitis.

a) **Outline your initial management strategy of this patient (14 marks)**

b) **What complications may arise due to severe acute pancreatitis? (6 marks)**

Aims

This core topic frequently requires assessment and admission to critical care, and several key features have changed relatively recently. A succinct answer regarding its management and the unique complications gives the impression of having managed this condition successfully on several occasions.

a) Management

i) Resuscitation
   - Early and aggressive fluid resuscitation. Regular clinical examination and blood tests: FBC, U&E, LFTs, clotting, amylase, lipase, ABG
   - Regular assessment for signs of deterioration. Consider use of scoring systems (e.g. Ranson, Imrie, APACHE II)
   - Awareness of ↑ risk of developing multi-organ dysfunction syndrome and local complications: age (>70years), BMI (>30kg/m²), evidence of pleural effusions or pancreatic necrosis, high Ranson score
   - Radiological scanning: ultrasound abdomen, CT abdomen (gold-standard post-adequate resuscitation) to assess presence of local complications
   - Analgesia: thoracic epidural will provide excellent analgesia; awareness for potential coagulopathy development must be accounted for

ii) Antibiotics
   - Prophylactic antibiotics are not routinely prescribed in necrotizing pancreatitis
   - If an infected abscess is found post fine-needle aspiration, antibiotics are prescribed according to local guidelines

iii) Nutrition
   - Early enteral feeding (e.g. naso-jejunal route) is encouraged to maintain good calorific intake
   - No advantages for routine TPN use; advocated if failure of enteral nutrition after one week
   - Maintenance of strict glycaemic control is important

iv) Surgery
   - CT-guided fine-needle aspiration is gold standard for detecting infected necrotic pancreas
   - If evidence of retroperitoneal gas on CT, broad-spectrum antibiotics and surgical drainage or debridement are indicated. Delayed surgery (>2 weeks) associated with ↑ survival and allows demarcation of necrotic pancreas and optimal tissue preservation

v) Gallstone-Induced Pancreatitis
   - If obstructive jaundice present, ERCP is indicated to remove common bile duct stones
   - Coagulation should be corrected prior to the procedure

vi) Critical Care Bundles
   • Use of known critical care bundles (e.g. glycaemic control, thromboembolism prophylaxis, gut protection, lung protective ventilation strategies to prevent acute lung injury)
   • If septic, patients are managed according to Surviving Sepsis Campaign guidelines

b) Complications

- Clinical factors (e.g. pain, persistent pyrexia, nausea and vomiting, and a palpable mass, together with raised inflammatory markers) often indicate the presence of an abscess or pseudocyst
- Abscess: may be a delayed presentation (e.g. 3–4 weeks post onset of disease). Risk is minimized by early scanning (i.e. CT or ultrasound). Treatment is percutaneous drainage or surgery
- Pseudocyst: intervention required only if significant symptoms (as above). Treatment is by endoscopic drainage or percutaneous aspiration and catheter drainage
- Infected necrosis requires urgent surgery; if sterile, supportive treatment is indicated
- Intra-abdominal hypertension: serial pressures to determine need for decompression
- Haemorrhage: due to rupture of pseudo-aneurysm of the splenic artery

Notes

References

Nathens AB, Curtis JR, Beale RJ, *et al.* Management of the critically ill patient with severe acute pancreatitis. *Critical Care Medicine*, **32**: 2524–36, 2004

Waldmann C. Pancreatitis. In: Waldmann C, Soni N, Rhodes A, eds. *Oxford Desk Reference: Critical Care*. Oxford University Press, 2008; 338–9

Young SP, Thompson JP. Severe acute pancreatitis. *Continuing Education in Anaesthesia, Critical Care & Pain*, **8**: 2008, 125–8

Q20 Percutaneous Tracheostomy

a) **List the indications for performing a tracheostomy (6 marks)**

b) **List the advantages and disadvantages of a percutaneous technique compared with the surgical alternative (7 marks)**

c) **List the relative contraindications for a percutaneous technique (7 marks)**

Aims

Clinicians must understand the benefits and risks of performing the procedure. Most trainees will have experience in tracheostomy insertion and subsequent management.

a) Indications for Tracheostomy

- To provide an airway during and after surgical procedures (e.g. craniofacial, oropharyngeal, laryngeal, or neck dissection surgery)
- To aid weaning from mechanical ventilation
- To facilitate suction of pulmonary secretions and prevent aspiration or LRTI
- To bypass upper airway obstruction, i.e. 2° to tumour, inflammation, infection, goitre
- Long-term respiratory support, i.e. neuromuscular disorders

b) Percutaneous Tracheostomy

i) Advantages
   - Relatively quick in experienced hands
   - Avoids need for transfer of unstable intubated patients from the ITU
   - Does not require involvement of surgeons to perform the procedure

ii) Disadvantages
   - Suboptimal conditions for management of bleeding, especially if major vessel injured
   - Blind techniques can be incorrectly positioned
   - Tracheal ring fracture has been described post dilatation
   - Late tracheal stenosis can occur, as for surgical tracheostomy
   - Lack of surgical dissection can increase risk of vascular or thyroid injury, especially in difficult patients (e.g. previous neck surgery, obesity, reduced neck movement)

c) Relative Contraindications for Performing Percutaneous Techniques

- <12 years old
- Coagulopathy
- Evidence of localized infection
- Local malignancy
- Unstable cervical spine fracture
- Difficult palpable anatomy (e.g. high BMI)
- Gross anatomical distortion (e.g. due to goitre)
- Previous neck surgery including tracheostomy
- Previous radiotherapy to the neck region
- Extensive burns to the neck
- High ventilatory support, i.e. PEEP >15, FiO_2 >60%

Notes

_____

_____

_____

_____

_____

_____

_____

_____

_____

_____

References

Delaney A, Bagshaw SM, Nalos M. Percutaneous dilatational tracheostomy versus surgical tracheostomy in critically ill patients: a systematic review and meta-analysis. *Critical Care*, **10**: R55, 2006

Freeman BD, Isabella K, Lin N, Buchman TG. A meta-analysis of prospective trials comparing percutaneous and surgical tracheostomy in critically ill patients. *Chest*, **118**: 1412–18, 2000

Griffiths J, Barber VS, Morgan L, Young JD. Systematic review and meta-analysis of studies of the timing of tracheostomy in adult patients undergoing artificial ventilation. *British Medical Journal*, **330**: 1243, 2005

Q21 **Rhabdomyolysis**

You are called to assess a 24-year-old woman with a history of intravenous drug abuse who was found collapsed at home. Her serum potassium level is 7.4mmol/L and her CK is 36,000 U/L. You notice that her urine is very dark in colour.

a) What is the most appropriate diagnosis in this patient? (1 mark)

b) Describe your immediate management of her life-threatening hyperkalaemia (5 marks)

c) Outline potential complications arising from this diagnosis (6 marks)

d) What further management would you institute for this patient? (8 marks)

Aims

This question aims to assess your ability to manage a life-threatening emergency. Rhabdomyolysis is a rare but serious complication of muscle necrosis, and knowledge of its treatment will suffice even if you have not seen a case in your unit.

a) Diagnosis
- Rhabdomyolysis

b) Hyperkalaemia
- Airway, breathing and 100% O_2 administration, circulation, and call for help
- Obtain IV access and connect ECG, NIBP, and pulse oximetry if not already done
- Myocardial membrane stabilization: give 10mL 10% calcium gluconate IV over 10min
- Encourage intracellular shift of K^+
  - 10 IU Actrapid® insulin in 50mL 50% dextrose
  - 5mg nebulized salbutamol
  - 50–100mmol sodium bicarbonate
- Increase K^+ elimination:
  - 20–250mg IV furosemide
  - Haemodialysis
- GI binding: sodium polystyrene sulphonate 30g PO/PR; then 15g TDS

c) Complications
i) Hyperkalaemia
  - This is the most prominent early complication, potentially leading to cardiac arrest (especially in combination with acidosis and hypocalcaemia)
ii) Compartment Syndrome
  - Fluid sequestration, oedema, and impaired compartment perfusion lead to ischaemia and nerve damage
iii) Acute Renal Failure
  - This is due to:
    - renal vasoconstriction
    - hypovolaemia
    - mechanical obstruction by intraluminal cast formation
    - direct cytotoxicity from myoglobin haem moieties

- ◆ myoglobin metabolism by-products releasing free radicals, which further exacerbate renal ischaemia
iv) Disseminated Intravascular Coagulation (DIC)
  - Commonly >72 hours post injury
v) Hypercalcaemia
  - Release of calcium into the intravascular compartment during the recovery phase may occur following accumulation at the time of muscle injury

d) Management of Rhabdomyolysis

- Admission to HDU or ICU for invasive cardiovascular monitoring and treatment
- Large-volume isotonic IV fluid therapy; aim for urine output of 200–300mL/hr
- Serial CK measurements to determine peak level
- If evidence of compartment syndrome, surgical fasciotomies may be required
- IV sodium bicarbonate titrated to urinary pH >6.5 to correct acidosis, reduce risk of hyperkalaemia, and increase urinary pH, thus preventing precipitation and degradation of myoglobin in the renal tubules
- IV mannitol: test dose 200mg/kg over 3–5min; then 10mL/hr
  - ◆ To ↑ renal blood flow and glomerular filtration rate
  - ◆ To ↓ muscle swelling and therefore risk of compartment syndrome
  - ◆ To promote diuresis and prevent precipitation of obstructive tubular casts
  - ◆ To serve as a free-radical scavenger
- Despite its use in the standard treatment of rhabdomyolysis, there is no clinical evidence that sodium bicarbonate or mannitol results in improved morbidity or mortality in these patients
- Consider renal replacement therapy in established acute renal failure where metabolic derangements are severe, or rarely in fluid overload
- Free-radical scavengers, antioxidants, and dantrolene have all been used as part of clinical trials but are as yet unproven

Notes

....

....

....

....

....

....

....

....

....

Reference

Stevens P. Rhabdomyolysis. In: Waldmann C, Soni N, Rhodes A, eds. *Oxford Desk Reference: Critical Care*. Oxford University Press, 2008; 502–3

Q22 Sepsis: 24 Hour Bundle

A 45-year-old man was admitted to ICU for treatment of deteriorating respiratory function and septic shock secondary to bilateral pneumonia.

a) **Define bundles of care in ICU and their aims (3 marks)**

b) **Following initial resuscitation of this patient, outline the important aspects of the longer-term sepsis bundle of care (17 marks)**

Aims

Following on from the acute management of sepsis, this question examines the extended care of a patient with defined septic shock whilst also exploring the broader areas of ICU management logistics and their aims.

a) Care Bundles

i) Definition
- A group of interventions related to a disease process that, when executed together, result in better outcomes than when implemented individually

ii) Aim
- To ensure that all patients receive the best treatment, based on evidence or logic, 100% of the time

b) Sepsis Bundle of Care (24 hours)

- This is the bundle of care that it is recommended and should be implemented within 24 hours of admitting a septic patient to ICU

i) Ventilator/Lung Management
- Tidal volume: 6mL/kg
- Upper limit plateau pressure: $\leq 30cmH_2O$
- Aim for PaO_2: >8kPa
- Permissive hypercapnia
- Use of optimal PEEP
- Other interventions which improve oxygenation, but have no proven effect on mortality rates, include inverse-ratio ventilation, conservative fluid strategy, prone position, nitric oxide, ECMO

ii) Glycaemic Control
- Monitor and treat hyperglycemia with an insulin/glucose infusion
- The Van den Berghe single-centre study suggested that outcome is improved with tight blood glucose control of 4–6mmol/L, but this has not been ratified and there is concern about the incidence of hypoglycaemia. The suggested range is now 4–8mmol/L

iii) Activated Protein C
- Consider in sepsis-induced organ dysfunction at high risk of death, i.e. where failure of two or more organs is present
- Consider pre-existing contraindications to activated protein C

iv) Steroids
- Short synacthen test not performed routinely. Suggested if evidence of steroid deficiency, i.e. previous panhypopituitarism, taking oral steroids, or bronchospasm
- Total hydrocortisone dose ≤300mg/day. Aim to stop as soon as possible

- Avoid steroids in septic shock unless patients are unresponsive to fluid resuscitation or vasopressors (grade 2C evidence)

v) DVT Prophylaxis:
- Unfractionated heparin or low molecular weight heparin should be prescribed in all patients according to local guidelines
- Use mechanical prophylactic devices where heparin is contraindicated

vi) Early Enteral Nutrition
- Supported to maintain healthy gut flora, mesenteric blood flow, calorie supplementation, and patency of bowel mucosa

vii) Stress Ulcer Prophylaxis
- H$_2$ blockers or PPIs: weigh benefits against risk of ventilator-associated pneumonia

viii) Other
- Selective decontamination of the gut: evidence currently split
- Use of vasopressin or terlipressin as an alternative vasopressor
- Laparostomy: management of intra-abdominal sepsis and compartment syndrome is increasingly being adopted
- CVVH vs intermittent haemodialysis: equivalent evidence (CVVH optimal in haemodynamically unstable patients)

Notes

References

Bernard GR, Vincent JL, Laterre PF, et al. Efficacy and safety of recombinant human activated protein C for severe sepsis. New England Journal of Medicine, **344**: 699–709, 2001

Lipiner-Friedman D, Sprung CL, Laterre PF, et al. Adrenal function in sepsis: the retrospective Corticus cohort study. Critical Care Medicine, **35**: 1012–18, 2007

Van den Berghe G, Wilmer A, Milants I, et al. Intensive insulin therapy in mixed medical/surgical intensive care units: benefit versus harm. Diabetes, **55**: 3151–9, 2006

Van den Berghe G, Wouters P, Weekers F, et al. Intensive insulin therapy in the critically ill patients. New England Journal of Medicine, **345**: 1359–67, 2001

Q23 Sepsis: 6 Hour Bundle

a) **Define the systemic inflammatory response syndrome (SIRS), sepsis, severe sepsis, and septic shock (4 marks)**

b) **Discuss key points in the immediate management of a septic patient, including early critical care interventions (16 marks)**

Aims

As this question involves both a core topic and a well-publicized document it should be easy to answer, but it is also easy to stray from the stem and lose marks and precious time. Read the question carefully: discussion is for the *immediate* management.

a) Definitions

- **SIRS**: two or more of the following:
    - body temperature <36°C or >38°C
    - HR >90bpm
    - RR >20/min
    - WBC <4 × 10^{9}cells/L or >12 × 10^9 cells/L
- **Sepsis**: SIRS + systemic manifestations of infection
- **Severe sepsis**: sepsis + evidence of acute organ dysfunction
- **Septic shock**: sepsis-induced hypotension despite adequate fluid resuscitation

b) Sepsis Management

- Outlined in Surviving Sepsis Campaign (SSC) guidelines: evidence-based recommendations for management of severe sepsis and septic shock

i) Resuscitation
    - Airway, breathing, and circulation
    - Targeted early goal-directed therapy within 6 hours of presentation to ↓ mortality at 28 days. Aim to achieve:
        - CVP 8–12mmHg
        - MAP >65mmHg
        - Urine output >0.5mL/kg/hr
        - Svo_2 ≥70 % (or mixed venous oxygen sats ≥65%)

ii) Microbiology
    - Two or more blood cultures (at least one percutaneous) before starting antibiotics
    - PCR-based assay: used to detect presence of micro-organisms to provide an accurate result within 2 hours
    - Begin broad-spectrum antibiotic therapy within 1 hour of onset of sepsis
    - Identify possible sources of infection (e.g. collections) and drain surgically or radiologically as quickly as possible
    - Remove potentially infected vascular access devices
    - Reassess daily as results and site become obvious, i.e. 48–72 hours
    - Monotherapy for 7–10 days has been shown to be most effective

iii) Fluid Therapy
    - Target CVP ≥8mmHg (≥12mmHg if IPPV)
    - Use fluid challenge technique
    - Large dextrans are associated with an increase in ARF and are best avoided

iv) Cardiovascular Support
- Vasopressors: to restore resting tone in arterial vascular bed
- Inotropes: to increase force of cardiac contraction
- Maintain MAP ≥65mmHg
- Centrally administered noradrenaline is the initial vasopressor of choice (may add vasopressin or terlipressin if noradrenaline-resistant hypotension)
- Dobutamine and adrenaline are used where myocardial dysfunction is evident, i.e. septic cardiomyopathy, pre-existing cardiac failure, or low cardiac output states

vii) Blood Products
- Transfuse only if Hb <7.0g/dL (<9.0 if coexisting IHD)
- Transfuse platelets if count <5 × 10^9/L, if 5–30 × 10^9/L and significant bleeding risk, or >50 × 10^9/L if invasive procedures or surgery required

Notes

....

....

....

....

....

....

....

....

....

....

....

....

References

Kumar A, Roberts D, Wood KE, *et al.* Duration of hypotension before initiation of effective antimicrobial therapy is the critical determinant of survival in human septic shock. *Critical Care Medicine*, **34**: 1589–96, 2006

Peters RP, van Agtmael, MA, Danner SA, Savelkoul EH, Vandenbroucke-Grauls CM. New developments in the diagnosis of bloodstream infections. *Lancet Infectious Diseases*, **4**: 751–60, 2004

Rivers E, Nguyen B, Havstad S, *et al.* Early goal-directed therapy in the treatment of severe sepsis and septic shock. *New England Journal of Medicine*, **345**: 1368–77, 2001

http://www.survivingsepsis.org/ (accessed 3 March 2010)

Q24 Tetanus

You are asked to provide an airway assessment of a 45-year-old builder who has presented to the Emergency Department with muscle spasms and difficulty in opening his mouth.

a) What is the most likely diagnosis? (1 mark)

b) Describe the pathophysiology of this disease (6 marks)

c) List the relevant features that may be found at examination (5 marks)

d) Outline your management plan for this patient (8 marks)

a) Diagnosis

- Tetanus

b) Pathophysiology

- *Clostridium tetani*: an anaerobic Gram –ve bacterium which produces a highly potent toxin
- Passage from soil, dust, animal or human faeces via contamination by bacterial spores of an open wound or abrasion
- On entry to the body, the bacillus releases tetanospasmin which cleaves synaptobrevin (the membrane protein vital for neurotransmitter release)
- Neurotransmitter release from presynaptic GABA-ergic and glycinergic inhibitory interneurons is inhibited
- Results in uncontrolled motor neuron activity with increased muscle tone and spasm, and an uninhibited sympathetic nervous system with CVS instability
- The disease course may be prolonged because of irreversible neuronal binding of neurotoxin

c) Examination

- Trismus: provoked by placing a wooden spatula in the mouth (patient bites down)
- Facial muscle spasm (risus sardonicus)
- Truncal muscle spasms (opisthotomus)
- Airway and respiratory compromise (laryngospasm may be potentially fatal)
- 'Autonomic storm': tachycardia, hypertension, sweating, pyrexia with periods of bradycardia, hypotension, and ultimately asystole
- Presence of an open wound (passage of infection)

d) Management

- Transfer to HDU or ICU, ideally a quiet dark side room
- i) Airway
    - If evidence of compromise, semi-elective intubation and ventilation. Caution: laryngoscopy may cause laryngospasm
    - Early tracheostomy to aid a prolonged respiratory wean
- ii) Spasm Control
    - High-dose IV benzodiazepines for muscular spasm (e.g. midazolam, diazepam)
    - Opiates (e.g. remifentanil, morphine)
    - Consider neuromuscular blocking drugs if severe disease
    - Magnesium sulphate, clonidine, and atropine: to aid CVS stability

- Other drugs that have been used: propofol, phenobarbitol, chlorpromazine, baclofen, and dantrolene

iii) Specific Treatment
- Human tetanus immunoglobulin infusion (5000–10000 units): one dose
  - intrathecal human immunoglobulin: ↓ disease progression and severity
- Tetanus antitoxin: subcutaneous administration
- Immunization with tetanus toxoid (in the recovery stage)
- Washing and surgical debridement of open wound
- Consider antibiotics if evidence of a wound infection (e.g. metronidazole)

iv) ICU Therapy
- Multidisciplinary support
- Early enteral feeding to promote nutrition
- Ventilator care bundles
- Thromboprophylaxis
- Monitoring for rhabdomyolysis (common after prolonged spasms)

Notes

References

Taylor AM. Tetanus. *Continuing Education in Anaesthesia, Critical Care & Pain*, **6**: 101–4, 2005
Thwaites L. Tetanus. In: Waldmann C, Soni N, Rhodes A, eds. *Oxford Desk Reference: Critical Care*. Oxford University Press, 2008; 378–9

Q25 Thyroid Storm

You are asked to urgently review an unwell 43-year-old woman in the Emergency Department with tachyarrhythmias and agitation. She is known to suffer from Graves' disease.

a) What is the most likely diagnosis? (1 mark)

b) Outline appropriate investigations and what you would expect to find (7 marks)

c) Describe your immediate management of this patient (12 marks)

Aims

This question explores how you would manage a key clinical problem including background understanding of the disease and relevant investigations, knowledge which you may not have been using regularly since house jobs. Background reading of core medical topics provides you with the ability to answer this and similar questions confidently.

a) Diagnosis

- Thyroid crisis

b) Investigations

i) Blood Tests
- FBC: raised WCC
- U&E: hypokalaemia, hypomagnesaemia, hypercalcaemia, hyperglycaemia
- TFTs: $\downarrow$ TSH, $\uparrow$ T_3 and T_4
- LFTs: $\uparrow$ ALT, AST, ALP, bilirubin
- ABG: mixed respiratory and metabolic acidosis
- Peripheral blood cultures

ii) Other Investigations
- ECG: arrhythmias, evidence of LVH
- CXR: cardiomegaly, pulmonary oedema

c) Immediate Management

- Medical emergency: treatment should not be delayed for biochemical confirmation if suspected
- ABC approach and 100% humidified oxygen
- Intubate and ventilate if severe cardiorespiratory compromise
- Fluid resuscitation: IV crystalloid therapy
- Correct electrolyte abnormalities (e.g. K^+, Mg^{2+})
- Active cooling: fluids, cold blankets, bladder irrigation
- Invasive cardiovascular monitoring
- Transfer to HDU or ICU
- Broad-spectrum antibiotics if infection suspected as trigger

i) Drugs

Corticosteroids
- Hydrocortisone 100mg IV QDS to correct deficit caused by thyrotoxicosis and decrease the peripheral conversion of T_4 to T_3

Drugs that alter thyroid hormone metabolism
- IV β-blockers: ↓ conversion of T_4 to T_3, ↓ catecholamine hypersensitivity, and block peripheral thyroid hormone effects
  - Propranolol 0.5mg increments to maximum 10mg, metoprolol 2–5mg increments to maximum 20mg, or esmolol 0.25–0.5mg/kg; then infusion 0.05–0.2mg/kg/min
- Carbimazole: blocks thyroid hormone synthesis, 60–120mg PO/NG/PR
- Propylthiouracil: blocks thyroxine synthesis and conversion of T_4 to T_3; 200mg 4 hourly PO/NG/PR
- Potassium iodide: blocks synthesis and release of thyroid hormones; 0.3mL Lugol's iodine diluted to 50mL TDS NG/PR given 1 hour before propylthiouracil
- Anti-arrhythmics: amiodarone, digoxin
- Other therapies: dantrolene if hyperpyrexial; reserpine or guanethidine if propranolol resistant; plasmapheresis

Notes

....

....

....

....

....

....

....

....

....

....

....

Reference

Philips B, Gordon S. Thyroid emergencies: thyroid crisis/thyrotoxic storm. In: Waldmann C, Soni N, Rhodes A, eds. *Oxford Desk Reference: Critical Care*. Oxford University Press, 2008; 432–3

Q26 Transoesophageal Echocardiography

a) **What are the indications for performing transoesophageal echocardiography (TOE)? (8 marks)**

b) **List potential complications of this procedure (6 marks)**

c) **Outline specific information that may be obtained during a TOE, including potential benefits to the patient (6 marks)**

Aims

Echocardiography is currently undergoing a renaissance in both theatre and critical care. Development of operator skills and advances in technology allow better-quality images which rapidly provide real-time evidence of cardiac filling and function. An increasing evidence base supporting its use in both these scenarios is evolving.

a) Indications for TOE

i) Preoperative
  - Assessment of cardiac function in patients whereby transthoracic imaging is not feasible (e.g. obesity, severe COPD)
  - Assessment of cardiac valves for the presence of vegetations in sepsis
  - Diagnosis of acute aortic dissection

ii) Perioperative
  - Assessment of cardiac structural function post cardiac surgery:
    - Post bypass cardiac contractility
    - Post valve repair or replacement cardiac function
    - Post surgery for hypertrophic obstructive cardiomyopathy or cardiac aneurysm repair
  - Assessment of LV function in sudden cardiac collapse where an explanation is unclear and response to resuscitation is poor
  - Assessment of suspected acute embolic phenomenon
  - Cardiac response to surgical interventions because of the ability to leave the probe *in situ* perioperatively allowing temporal comparisons
  - Monitoring for cardiac ischaemia in patients at high risk of cardiac events undergoing non-cardiac surgery
  - Detection of air emboli in neurosurgery

iii) Postoperative
  - Placement of cardiac assist devices, i.e. ventricular assist device
  - Assessment of pericardial collections, especially in the posterior location

b) Complications

  - Sore throat
  - Dental injury
  - Displacement of airway device
  - Vocal cord damage
  - Thermal injury
  - GI tract bleeding
  - Oesophageal perforation (rare in absence of pre-existing oesophageal disease)

- Arrhythmias
- Infection
- Overall, risks appear to be lower than for upper GI endoscopy

c) Information Gained from a TOE

- Heart rate and rhythm
- Assessment of filling status and response to filling
- Ventricular contractility
- Cardiac output
- Presence of regional wall motion abnormalities and response to treatment
- Function and flow across intracardiac valves
- Presence of extracardiac collections (pericardial, pleural)
- Volume of intracardiac air, emboli
- Detailed images of the posterior structures of the heart, i.e. aorta and atria

Notes

Q27 Transfusion-Related Acute Lung Injury

You are called to assess a 76-year-old man on ICU whose respiratory parameters on arterial blood sampling are worsening. He is 4 hours post emergency repair of a ruptured abdominal aortic aneurysm, and intraoperatively underwent massive transfusion to achieve stability.

a) What is the most likely cause of his deterioration? (3 marks)

b) Discuss the proposed pathogenesis for developing this pathology (8 marks)

c) What management strategies exist for treatment? (9 marks)

Aims

Although well recognized as a potential complication following blood product administration, the pathogenesis behind transfusion-related acute lung injury (TRALI) is still not clear. Although it mimics ARDS, its clinical progression is very different and this question explores your background knowledge and management.

a) Cause
- Transfusion-related acute lung injury
- An acute onset of respiratory distress following administration of blood products, usually within hours (some definitions use 6 hours as a cut-off), after exclusion of all other possible explanations, with associated hypoxaemia and pulmonary infiltrates

b) Pathogenesis
- Proposed pathogenesis focuses around either immune or mechanical theories
- i) Immune
  - HLA and HNA antigens activate the innate immune system, resulting in an acute inflammatory response
  - Results in pulmonary leucostasis and release of pro-inflammatory mediators with subsequent increases in pulmonary capillary permeability and oedema
  - In 5–15% of patients, no antibody is found
  - Two-hit hypothesis used to explain this phenomenon:
    - First hit: severe illness causes increased concentration of neutrophils into the pulmonary circulation
    - Second hit: transfusion of HLA-rich blood causes activation of neutrophils resulting in a localized pro-inflammatory reaction
- ii) Mechanical
  - Microthrombi particulates within stored products are filtered out by the pulmonary microcirculation, resulting in vaso-occlusion and subsequent inflammation and oedema
  - Biologically active lipids possessing capabilities of activating neutrophil oxidase, which may subsequently cause damage to the pulmonary vascular endothelium, develop in stored blood products

c) Diagnosis and Management
- Diagnosis is based on confirming the presence of an acute lung injury and excluding other possible explanations or triggers
- Assess for presence of symptoms and signs consistent with ALI or ARDS
  - Increased work of breathing

- ◆ Hypotension
- ◆ Presence of pulmonary oedema
- ◆ Presence of pyrexia
- Look for signs of elevated venous pressure (raised CVP and PAOP)
  - ◆ If present indicates fluid overload, probably 2° to cardiac pump failure
- Upper airway obstruction, i.e. stridor or dysphonia
  - ◆ Possible anaphylaxis
- Systemic signs of high cardiac output
  - ◆ Potential diagnosis of sepsis and SIRS, possibly due to infection of blood products
- If none of the above present, consider TRALI
  - ◆ ABG: allows clinicians to distinguish between ALI and ARDS
  - ◆ Response of hypoxia to oxygenation
  - ◆ CXR: presence of bilateral pulmonary infiltrates
- Management is as for ARDS, aiming to ensure adequate oxygenation (aiming for PaO_2 >8kPa) with the minimum FiO_2 possible to limit O_2-induced ALI
- Fluid resuscitate to maintain adequate organ perfusion whilst attempting to avoid worsening of ALI
- Consider use of NIV or invasive ventilation with optimal PEEP to improve oxygenation
- Diagnosis of TRALI confirmed by acute onset of symptoms, followed by rapid resolution of signs and symptoms (usually within 96 hours)

Notes

Reference

Silliman CC, McLaughlin NJ. Transfusion-related acute lung injury. *Blood Reviews*, **20**: 139–59, 2006

Q28 **Vasopressin**

a) **How does vasopressin exert its physiological actions in the body? (10 marks)**

b) **Discuss current and potential uses for vasopressin in clinical practice (10 marks)**

Aims

Vasopressin is currently under assessment in several situations as a potential exogenous vasopressor. Its pharmacodynamics are different from those of traditional vasopressors, and there is an emerging evidence base regarding its use in clinical medicine.

a) Vasopressin Receptors

- G-protein coupled receptors with seven transmembrane-spanning domains
- i) V_1 Receptors
  - Vascular smooth muscle receptor found in the heart, kidneys, hepatocytes, bladder, spleen, platelets, and adipocytes
  - G_q protein-coupled activation of phospholipase C and release of intracellular Ca^{2+} mediates vascular vasoconstriction (exacerbated in hypovolaemia to maintain organ perfusion)
  - Vasodilatation of pulmonary and cerebral vessels is achieved by NO-mediated action
- ii) V_2 Receptors
  - Found on the distal convoluted tubules and collecting ducts of the kidney: they are essential for osmolality and plasma volume control
  - G_s protein-coupled activation of adenylcyclase leads to $\uparrow$ cAMP production, activation of aquaporin channels, $\uparrow$ H_2O reabsorption, and an antidiuretic effect
  - Also present on endothelial cells: stimulation releases von Willebrand factor (vWF) which plays an important role in platelet aggregation and binding where bleeding occurs
- iii) V_3 Receptors
  - G_q protein-coupled activation results in $\uparrow$ intracellular Ca^{2+}
  - Responsible for CNS action of vasopressin, i.e. acts as a neurotransmitter modulating control of memory, BP, core temperature, and release of pituitary hormones
- iv) Oxytocin Receptor (OTR)
  - Found in the endothelial cells of reproductive organs, vascular endothelium, and heart
  - Actions include uterine vasoconstriction, NO-mediated vasodilatation, and ANP release
- v) Purinergic Receptors (P_2R)
  - Found in cardiac endothelium and myocardium
  - Stimulation causes selective coronary vasodilatation and $\uparrow$ cardiac contractility

b) Clinical Uses for Vasopressin

- Cardiac arrest: ongoing research to demonstrate effectiveness as an alternative to adrenaline in patients with out-of-hospital asystolic cardiac arrest. Its vasoconstrictive efficacy in severe acidosis results in better coronary perfusion during cardiac resuscitation
- Diabetes insipidus (DI): intranasal or IV desmopressin is used to treat cranial DI (2° to TBI, SAH, neoplasms) and reduce polyuria
- Oesophageal varices: terlipressin (synthetic long-acting vasopressin analogue) decreases portal blood flow, hepatic venous pressure gradient, and also variceal pressure during haemorrhage

- Bleeding and coagulopathy: desmopressin (synthetic analogue of vasopressin) is used in mild forms of haemophilia A, von Willebrand disease (vWD), and conditions with impaired platelet function 2° to renal failure or drugs to increase efficiency of platelet activation and coagulation
- Shock: there are beneficial haemodynamic effects in septic shock unresponsive to conventional vasopressors
  - Used in both refractory haemorrhagic and anaphylactic shock where the response to fluids, blood, and catecholamines may be poor because of persistent acidosis, receptor downregulation, and NO-induced vasodilatation
- Neuroendocrine tumour resection: for treatment of catecholamine-resistant hypotension (e.g. post phaeochromocytoma removal)
- Organ donation: helps to preserve organ function, is less likely to cause metabolic acidosis and pulmonary hypertension, reduces inotrope requirement in brain-dead patients before surgery, and treats diabetes insipidus

Notes

References

Russell JA, Walley KR, Singer J, et al. Vasopressin versus norepinephrine infusion in patients with septic shock. New England Journal of Medicine, **358**: 877–87, 2008

Sharman A, Low J. Vasopressin and its role in critical care. Continuing Education in Anaesthesia, Critical Care & Pain, **8**: 134–7, 2008

Part 3 Anatomy and Regional Techniques

Q1 Ankle Block

A 45-year-old woman is having surgery for left hallux valgus correction.

a) **Describe the sensory innervation of the foot and ankle (8 marks)**

b) **List possible options for anaesthetising the foot for surgery (3 marks)**

c) **Describe how you would perform an ankle block (9 marks)**

Aims

This question remains a popular topic in the examination and should be easy to reproduce. Alternative techniques provide another way of providing similar effects with a different technique, and a structured approach is the best way of tackling this style of question.

a) Sensory Innervation of the Foot

i) Saphenous Nerve
  - Terminal branch of the femoral nerve
  - Enters the foot anterior to the medial malleolus, adjacent to the long saphenous vein
  - Supplies the medial border of the foot up to the ball of the great toe

ii) Posterior Tibial Nerve
  - Mixed motor and sensory terminal branch of the tibial nerve
  - Enters the foot posterior to the medial malleolus behind the posterior tibial artery
  - Divides into medial and lateral plantar nerves that supply the sole of the foot

iii) Sural nerve
  - Branch of the tibial nerve, arising below the popliteal fossa
  - Occasionally receives accessory input from the common peroneal nerve
  - Supplies the lateral border of the foot and the fifth toe
  - Enters the foot superficially and posterior to the lateral malleolus

iv) Deep Peroneal Nerve
  - Branch of the common peroneal nerve; lies just lateral to the dorsalis pedis artery
  - Enters the foot as terminal sensory branches, passing underneath the extensor retinaculum before dividing into medial and lateral branches
  - Lateral branch is motor to the extensor digitorum brevis
  - Medial branch supplies a small area over the dorsum of the foot (first web space)

v) Superficial Peroneal Nerve
  - Other branch of the common peroneal nerve
  - Becomes superficial in lower third of calf between peroneus tertius and brevis before dividing into medial and intermediate dorsal cutaneous nerves
  - Branches enter the foot by passing over the extensor retinaculum
  - Medial dorsal cutaneous nerve supplies the medial part of the dorsum of the foot and supplements first and second web spaces
  - Intermediate dorsal cutaneous nerve supplies the lateral dorsum and the third and fourth web spaces

b) Options for Blocking These Nerves During Surgery
  - Central (e.g. subarachnoid or epidural block)
  - Nerve root (e.g. lumbosacral plexus or paravertebral blockade)

- Nerve trunks (e.g. sciatic/femoral, popliteal fossa blocks)
- Ankle block

c) Ankle Block

- Standard preoperative assessment and procedural consent:
  - S   Sterile equipment
  - L   Light source
  - I   IV Access
  - M   Monitoring
  - R   Resuscitation equipment
  - A   Assistant trained in regional and general anaesthesia
  - G   Ability to convert to GA if required or appropriate

i)   Saphenous
  - Superficial and anterior to the medial malleolus, inject LA from the medial malleolus to the Achilles tendon subcutaneously, then anteriorly to the tibia

ii)   Posterior Tibial
  - Posterior to the medial malleolus, advance needle onto bone and then withdraw 1–2mm before injecting LA

iii)   Deep Peroneal
  - Lateral to dorsalis pedis artery on the dorsum of the foot; 3–5mL injected deep to the fascial plane

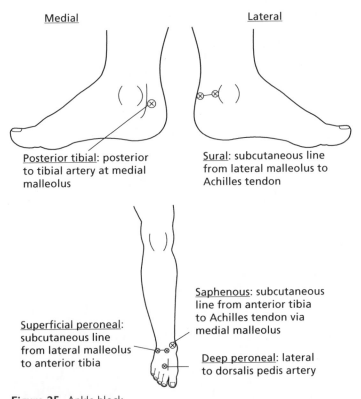

Figure labels:

Medial

Lateral

Posterior tibial: posterior to tibial artery at medial malleolus

Sural: subcutaneous line from lateral malleolus to Achilles tendon

Superficial peroneal: subcutaneous line from lateral malleolus to anterior tibia

Saphenous: subcutaneous line from anterior tibia to Achilles tendon via medial malleolus

Deep peroneal: lateral to dorsalis pedis artery

Figure 25. Ankle block

iv) Superficial Peroneal
- Division of the nerve is at a variable distance above the lateral malleolus making a single shot technically difficult
- Subcutaneous infiltration from the lateral malleolus to the anterior aspect of the tibia should block this nerve

v) Sural Nerve
- Linear blockade subcutaneously from the lateral malleolus to the Achilles tendon
- Use of a nerve stimulator will only be of benefit in locating mixed nerves, and ultrasound is increasingly being used to perform single-shot injection techniques rather than linear subcutaneous infiltration

Notes

Q2 Antecubital Fossa

a) **Describe the boundaries and contents of the antecubital fossa (10 marks)**
b) **List indications for vessel cannulation in this region (4 marks)**
c) **What complications may arise from cannulation of these vessels? (6 marks)**

Aims

A common area of anatomy for anaesthesia and critical care, the applied regional anatomy of the antecubital fossa is important not only for vascular access but also for nerve blockade of the forearm, especially with the advent of ultrasound-guided blocks.

a) Boundaries and Contents

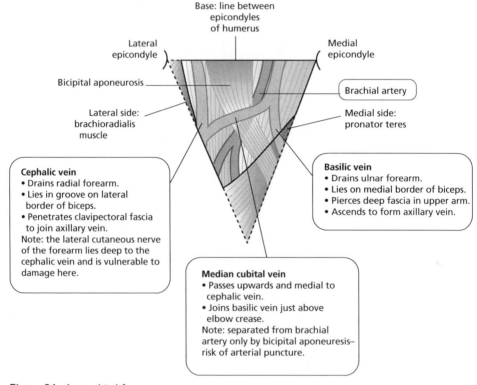

Figure 26. Antecubital fossa

i) Boundaries
- Medial: lateral border of pronator teres
- Lateral: medial border of brachioradialis
- Superior: horizontal line connecting medial and lateral epicondyles of humerus
- Roof: skin, superficial and deep fascia partially formed by the bicipital aponeurosis

- Floor: formed by the brachialis and supinator muscles overlying the capsule of the elbow joint

ii) Nerves
- Ulnar: continuation of the medial cord of the brachial plexus; enters the fossa medial to the brachial artery
- Lateral cutaneous of forearm (musculocutaneous): runs along radial border
- Medial cutaneous (medial cord of brachial plexus): runs along ulnar border
- Median: enters medial to the brachial artery, giving off articular branches to the elbow joint, and exits over pronator teres before giving off the anterior interosseus nerve
- Radial: located along lateral radial border; runs between brachioradialis and brachialis muscles. Not consistently found in the fossa

iii) Arteries
- Brachial artery: enters fossa between median nerve (medial) and biceps tendon (lateral). Lies deep to the bicipital aponeurosis. Bifurcates at apex to form superficial radial artery and deeper ulnar artery

iv) Veins
- Cephalic vein: ascends along the radial aspect of the forearm. Crosses in roof of fossa and ascends arm lateral to biceps to deltopectoral groove where it pierces fascia and joins axillary vein.
- Basilic vein: ascends the medial (ulnar) aspect of forearm and crosses in roof of fossa medial to the biceps. In the middle of the arm it pierces the biceps fascia and joins the brachial vein to form the axillary vein
- Median cubital vein: connects cephalic and basilic veins across the cubital fossa. Crosses the brachial artery separated only by the deep fascia

b) Indications

- Diagnostic: procedures such as venepuncture, administration of contrast during imaging procedures
- Therapeutic
  - insertion of IV cannulas for elective or emergency procedures, i.e. administration of GA or drug infusions
  - arterial or venous blood gas sampling
  - invasive blood pressure monitoring
  - insertion of peripheral long lines, i.e. PICC or Drum catheters for long-term antibiotic administration, feeding, or assessment of central venous pressures

c) Complications

i) Immediate
- Infiltration: incorrect position of needle or cannula tip outside lumen of vessel
- Extravasation: administration of fluid or drug into adjacent tissue with possible resultant injury (e.g. necrosis)
- Air embolization
- Incorrect vessel cannulated, i.e. artery instead of vein with potential for intra-arterial injection
- Nerve injury: more common during arterial line insertion because of the proximity of the median nerve and brachial artery
- Critical ischaemia to the distal forearm: the brachial artery is an end artery; complete occlusion could result from dissection or thrombus at line insertion site

ii) Late
- Infection
  - Research has shown that aseptic insertion of cannulas significantly reduces the incidence of bacteraemia in hospitalized patients
  - Similar work has looked at superficial infection at the insertion site with subsequent bacteraemia
  - Scoring systems: Visual Infusion Phlebitis (VIP) scores are routinely used to assess this; recommendations suggest that cannulas are recommended to remain *in situ* for no longer than three days
- Thrombophlebitis

Notes

....

....

....

....

....

....

....

....

....

....

....

Reference

The Multimedia Procedure Manual. Available online at: http://emprocedures.com/peripheralIV/introduction.htm (accessed 15 November 2009)

Q3 Central Neuraxial Blockade

You wish to insert a thoracic epidural as the primary perioperative mode of analgesia for a 76-year-old man undergoing an elective open anterior resection.

a) **List contraindications to performing central neuraxial blockade in this patient (6 marks)**

b) **What are the potential benefits (7 marks) and risks (7 marks) of performing an epidural in this case?**

Aims

This is a common procedure regularly performed in both elective and emergency surgery. Knowing when not to perform this procedure is a significant part of the technique. Understanding the pros and cons allows you to communicate these to the patient to help appreciate why you wish to perform this procedure. Updated evidence has been published recently in the NAP3 project.

a) Contraindications to Central Neuraxial Blockade

i) Absolute
- Patient refusal
- Local anaesthetic allergy
- Localized area of infection at insertion site
- Distorted anatomy likely to make insertion impossible

ii) Relative
- Thrombocytopenia (platelet count <80 × 10^9/L)
- Coagulopathy
  - acquired, e.g. sepsis, drugs (warfarin, heparin, antiplatelet agents)
  - congenital, e.g. factor VIII/IX deficiency, von Willebrand's disease
- Severe hypovolaemic state
- Severe cardiac valve lesions, e.g. stenoses (slow top-up epidural techniques are used)

b) Benefits and Risks

i) Epidural Benefits
- Gold-standard of analgesia for this type of surgery
- Reduction in the need for perioperative IV opioids
- Reduction in intraoperative blood loss
- Potential psychological and financial benefits; aiding speed of recovery and time to discharge
- Reduction in postoperative complications
  - Mortality: some studies exist to prove decrease in postoperative mortality rates
  - Wound infection rates (2° to superior tissue perfusion)
  - Myocardial infarction
  - Thromboembolic phenomena (e.g. DVT/PE)
  - Respiratory depression
  - Lower respiratory tract infection
  - Nausea and vomiting
- Earlier recovery of gut function and enteral feeding commencement
- Decreased time to extubation and shorter length of stay in ICU

ii) Risks

Early

- Hypotension or bradycardia (may progress to cardiovascular compromise and collapse)
- Nausea and vomiting (usually 2° to hypotension or opioids)
- Itching
- Shivering
- Failure to provide analgesia
- Unilateral block
- Subdural block
- Dural tap
- Intrathecal catheter: may lead to a high or total spinal
- Intravascular injection or infusion

Late

- Post dural puncture headache (less common at extremes of age)
- Urinary retention
- Nerve damage:
  - temporary or permanent neuropathy (sensory or motor deficit)
  - spinal cord ischaemia/damage
  - tetraplegia, paraplegia
- Vertebral canal haematoma
- Infection:
  - superficial
  - vertebral canal abscess
  - meningitis

Notes

Reference

Royal College of Anaesthetists. *National Audit of Major Complications of Central Neuraxial Block in the United Kingdom. Third National Audit Project of the Royal College of Anaesthetists (NAP3)*. London: Royal College of Anaesthetists, 2009

Q4 Coeliac Plexus

a) **List the indications for coeliac plexus blockade (6 marks)**

b) **Describe a technique for blocking this ganglion (7 marks)**

c) **What are the complications of a coeliac plexus block (7 marks)**

Aims

Most candidates are unlikely to have seen one of these blocks being performed. However, they remain very effective in certain cohorts, and good knowledge of regional anatomy allows many of the complications and side effects to be predicted.

a) Indications

- The block has both diagnostic and therapeutic uses
- i) Analgesic
  - Diagnosis of chronic pain syndrome (confirmation of sympathetic-mediated chronic pain syndromes by blockade of the plexus)
  - Chronic abdominal visceral pain, e.g. chronic pancreatitis (less effective than its malignant equivalent)
  - Acute pain, i.e. postoperative laparotomy patients (often in combination with intercostal nerve blocks)
- ii) Neurolytic
  - Malignancy: pancreatic carcinoma is the most common indication, although any of the abdominal viscera can be affected
  - Pain relief is classed as good in up to 90% of patients

b) Technique

- Usually performed as a day case; elderly or frail patients may require overnight admission
- Standard preoperative assessment and procedural consent
  - S   Sterile equipment
  - L   Light source
  - I   IV Access
  - M   Monitoring
  - R   Resuscitation equipment
  - A   Assistant trained in regional and general anaesthesia
  - G   Ability to convert to GA if required or appropriate
- Patient lies prone
- A 20G 10–15cm needle is inserted at the level of L1 just below the tip of the 12th rib
- X-ray screening in the AP and lateral views confirms the position of the needle as it advances to touch the body of L1
- The needle is withdrawn, angled anterior, and advanced a further 2–3cm to lie just anterior to the abdominal aorta
- Position is confirmed with the use of radio-opaque contrast
- Endoscopic ultrasound-guided blocks are now being advocated as easier to perform, with lower risks of spinal and visceral injury, and equal efficacy

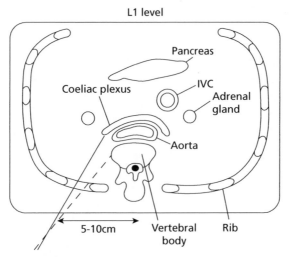

Figure 27. Coeliac plexus block

c) Complications

i) Immediate
  - Nerve injury
  - Vascular injury to IVC or abdominal aorta
  - Intravascular injection (risk reduced with X-ray guidance)
  - Abdominal visceral puncture (renal most likely)
  - Incorrect injection site:
    - subarachnoid
    - epidural
    - intramuscular injection (e.g. psoas)

ii) Early
  - Anterior spinal artery syndrome, especially with phenol
  - Hypotension due to splanchnic circulatory vasodilation
  - Diarrhoea
  - Acute pancreatitis
  - Peritonitis secondary to visceral puncture (especially bowel)
  - Lumbar plexus irritation due to spread of neurolytic solutions
  - Intoxication in alcohol-based injections in frail or elderly patients

iii) Late
  - Sexual dysfunction (injected solution spreads to the sympathetic chain bilaterally)
  - Recurrence of pain: often duration of block only 6 months
  - Neuro-ablative blocks can be associated with painful neuroma formation, chronic altered sensation, and a neuropathic pain picture

Notes

_____

_____

_____

_____

_____

_____

_____

_____

_____

_____

_____

_____

References

Michaels AJ, Draganov PV. Endoscopic ultrasonography guided celiac plexus neurolysis and celiac plexus block in the management of pain due to pancreatic cancer and chronic pancreatitis. _World Journal of Gastroenterology_, **13**: 3575–80, 2007

http://www.medicine.ox.ac.uk/bandolier/booth/painpag/Chronrev/Cancer/CP083.html (accessed 2 December 2009)

Q5 Eye Blocks

a) **Describe the innervation of the eye (8 marks)**
b) **Describe techniques for performing i) a retrobulbar block (6 marks) and ii) a peribulbar block (6 marks)**

Aims

Exposure to regional blocks in ophthalmics is becoming rarer for trainees, especially with the advent of the sub-Tenon's block. Despite these changes in practice, peri and retrobulbar procedures remain popular in the examination, and a clear understanding of the differences between the two is paramount.

a) Innervation of the Eye

- The globe receives motor, sensory, and autonomic innervation from nerve trunks which enter via the back of the orbit through the optic canal and the superior and inferior orbital fissures

i) Motor
- Extra-ocular: enters via the superior orbital fissure. Remember (LR6 SO4)3
  - Superior oblique: cranial nerve IV (trochlear)
  - Lateral rectus: cranial nerve VI (abducens)
  - Remaining extra-ocular muscles including levator palpebrae superioris: cranial nerve III (oculomotor)

ii) Autonomic
- Autonomic innervation of the papillary muscles allows the diameter of the pupil to alter the amount of light conveyed onto the retina
- Contraction of the dilator papillary muscles is triggered by sympathetic impulses along the short and long ciliary nerves originating in the superior cervical ganglion (mydriasis)
- These axons run along the internal carotid artery
- Meiosis is triggered by parasympathetic fibres which run from the Edinger–Westphal nucleus in the oculomotor nerve, synapsing in the ciliary ganglion. From here, short post-ganglionic ciliary nerves innervate the circular constrictor muscle

iii) Sensory
- Branches of the trigeminal nerve supply the skin of the eyelids and the conjunctiva
- The ophthalmic division gives lacrimal, nasociliary, and frontal nerves (via superior orbital fissure)
- The maxillary division gives the infra-orbital nerve (via inferior orbital fissure)
- Special sensory: the greater petrosal nerve branches from the facial nerve at the geniculate ganglion to supply parasympathetic autonomic innervation to the pterygopalatine ganglion which is responsible for lacrimation from the lacrimal gland
- The optic nerve conveys impulses from the retina to the optic chiasm

b) Techniques

i) Retrobulbar Block
- Intraconal injection with a 40mm 25G needle
- Percutaneous or transconjunctival techniques are both possible
- Inferotemporal quadrant is the chosen area because of a relative deficiency of blood vessels

- Check axial length of globe: contraindicated where axial length >26mm
- Injection point is in line with the lateral edge of the iris
- Advance the needle 1cm; then angle it superomedially, piercing the muscle cone
- The eye will 'bob' downwards upon penetration of the cone
- Aspirate and inject 4–5mL of LA
- Less popular because of a higher incidence of globe perforation and neurovascular injury
- Often requires a supplemental facial nerve block for orbicularis oculi

ii) Peribulbar block
- Extraconal injection with a larger dose of LA, usually 5–10mL
- Shorter needle as aim is not to pass the equator of the globe
- Injection point as for retrobulbar technique
- Advance the needle posteriorly to touch the posterior wall of the orbit
- Aspirate and inject 5–10ml of LA
- May require a medial injection of 2–5ml of LA performed at the medial caruncle
- Additional facial nerve blockade is not usually required

Notes

Q6 Fascia Iliaca Block

a) **Outline i) the indications and ii) the contraindications to performing a fascia iliaca block (6 marks)**

b) **Describe techniques used in performing a fascia iliaca block (7 marks)**

c) **List the advantages and disadvantages of this block (7 marks)**

Aims

Even if you have not performed the fascia iliaca block, a good level of understanding will allow you to give an accurate description of how to perform the procedure and the relative indications. Its popularity is growing for management of hip surgery, and several techniques exist including catheter and ultrasound techniques.

a) Fascia Iliaca Block

i) Indications
- Analgesia for fracture of the femur at any point
- As an analgesic adjunct for hip surgery (except the dorsal aspect of hip which is supplied by the sciatic nerve)
- Surgery on the anteromedial aspect of the thigh (e.g. skin grafting)
- Knee arthroscopy (combined with sciatic nerve block or intra-articular analgesia)
- Total knee replacement (combined with sciatic nerve block)

ii) Contraindications
Absolute
- Patient refusal
- Local anaesthetic allergy
- Localized infection

Relative
- Systemic sepsis
- Coagulopathy
- Localized tumour-containing tissue
- Ipsilateral pelvic renal transplant
- Lower limb neurological deficit

b) Techniques

- Standard preoperative assessment and procedural consent
  S   Sterile equipment
  L   Light source
  I   IV access
  M Full monitoring
  R   Resuscitation equipment available
  A   Assistant trained in regional and general anaesthesia
  G   Ability to convert to GA if appropriate
- Patient is in the supine position
- Insertion point is described as 1cm below the junction of the lateral and middle third of the inguinal ligament (line between the anterior superior iliac spine and pubic tubercle)
- The plane can be identified when two clicks are felt as the block needle passes through the fascia lata followed by the fascia iliaca

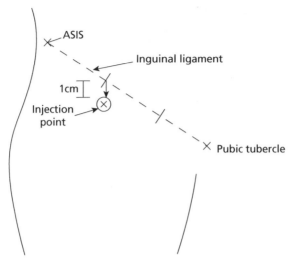

Figure 28. Fascia iliaca block: ASIS, anterior superior iliac spine

- After negative aspiration, either single-shot techniques (25–30mL local anaesthetic) or catheter techniques have been described
- Larger-volume techniques may achieve a block of the more cephalic branches of the lumbar plexus by tracking into the psoas fascial plane
- Ultrasound techniques to identify the correct plane and confirm spread of local anaesthetic are now popular and well described

c) Advantages and Disadvantages

i) Advantages
- No stimulator needle required, therefore more comfortable in an awake patient
- Supine block, patient does not need to move
- Can safely insert a catheter for post-operative analgesia
- More consistent block of both the lateral femoral cutaneous nerve of the thigh and femoral nerve compared with a '3-in-1' block
- Better anaesthesia and analgesia for hip surgery compared with a '3-in-1' block
- Lack of side effects seen with central neuraxial blockade

ii) Disadvantages
- Local anaesthetic often fails to block the higher branches of the lumbar plexus (especially with continuous catheter infusion techniques)
- Risk of visceral or peritoneal injury during insertion
- External iliac vessels are in relatively close proximity: care must be taken to avoid IV injection of LA

Notes

References

Farrugia D. The fascia iliaca block. *CPD Anaesthesia*, **9**: 109–13, 2007
http://www.usra.ca/upload/UIA/20071102052342/Fascia%20Iliaca%20Block.pdf (accessed 28 September 2009)

Q7 Femoral Nerve

You wish to perform a femoral nerve block on an 82-year-old woman for a right hemi-arthroplasty.

a) **Outline the motor and sensory distribution of the femoral nerve along its course (6 marks)**

b) **Describe a technique for performing a femoral nerve block (8 marks)**

c) **What complications may occur during this procedure? (6 marks)**

Aims

This is a core procedure in a variety of surgical settings. The applied anatomy of the femoral nerve and its neighbours is a common topic that should be relatively straightforward.

a) Anatomy

- The femoral nerve is the largest branch of the lumbar plexus
- The anterior primary rami of L2–4 divide into anterior and posterior divisions. The posterior divisions unite within the substance of the psoas major muscle to form the femoral nerve
- The femoral nerve leaves the lateral border of the psoas muscle and runs downwards to cross the inguinal ligament just lateral to the femoral vessels to enter the femoral triangle
- It lies lateral to the femoral canal and sheath and is separated from them by the fascia iliaca
- Branching of the femoral nerve to form an anterior and posterior branch, which quickly subdivide further, usually occurs below the inguinal ligament. There is considerable variation in the site at which this branching occurs, with the anterior branch occasionally branching directly from the lumbar plexus

i) Anterior Branch
- Supplies the skin over the front and medial thigh via the medial and intermediate cutaneous nerves of the thigh
- Provides the muscular branches to the sartorius and pectineus muscles

ii) Posterior Branch
Divides into three further branches
- The articular branch provides innervation to the hip and knee joints.
- The muscular branch supplies the quadriceps muscles.
- The largest terminal division, the saphenous nerve, runs through the adductor canal, and then becomes superficial and continues below the knee to supply skin along the medial aspect of the calf and occasionally the great toe

b) Technique

- Standard preoperative assessment and procedural consent
  S Sterile equipment
  L Light source
  I IV Access
  M Full monitoring
  R Resuscitation equipment available
  A Assistant trained in regional and general anaesthesia
  G Ability to convert to GA if block appropriate

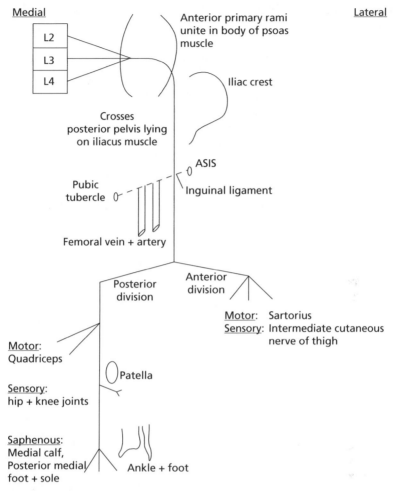

Figure 29. Femoral nerve: ASIS, anterior superior iliac spine

- Patient lies supine with the leg marked, hip and knee joints neutral
- LA to skin if performed awake. The puncture site lies approximately 1cm lateral to the femoral pulse and 1cm below the inguinal ligament
- A short peripheral nerve stimulator needle is attached to a peripheral nerve stimulator and advanced at a 45° rostral angle to a depth of 1–3cm. Occasionally the nerve lies at a depth >4cm, although this is unusual. Two clicks may be felt as the needle passes first through the fascia lata and then the fascia iliaca
- Correct placement is indicated by visible and palpable contraction of the quadriceps muscle, indicated by movement of the patella. If contraction of the sartorius is observed, the needle should be repositioned more laterally
- After negative aspiration, a volume of 15–20mL of LA is injected without resistance, whilst aspirating regularly to confirm extravascular placement
- Ultrasound techniques allow accurate identification of the nerve and visualization of LA within the fascia iliaca plane to produce the block

- Can be a single-shot technique or modified equipment allows insertion of a catheter for continuous postoperative infusions

c) Complications

i) Immediate
- Intravascular injection and subsequent local anaesthetic toxicity
- Intraneural injection
- Failure of block

ii) Early
- Haematoma formation
- Motor: weak hip flexion
- Proximal migration of local solution can cause blockade of more proximal branches of the lumbar plexus
- Superficial infection: more likely with indwelling catheters *in situ* >48 hours

iii) Late
- Compression neuropathy
- Sensory loss
- Pain
- Weakness of quadriceps

Notes

References

http://www.neuraxiom.com/html/femoral.php (accessed 13 October 2009)
http://www.usra.ca/sb_femoral (accessed 13 October 2009)

Q8 Infraclavicular Brachial Plexus Block

A 60-year-old woman is listed for an open reduction and internal fixation of a fractured distal humerus. She has been consented for an infraclavicular brachial plexus block.

a) Describe the blind midclavicular approach for performing this block (11 marks)

b) What response may be elicited when the posterior cord, lateral cord, medial cord, and subscapular nerve is stimulated? (6 marks)

c) List the complications of this technique (3 marks)

Aims

The brachial plexus is a common theme in examinations and should be core knowledge. There are a variety of approaches with individual merits, and you should be able to compare and contrast these even if you have not seen or done them. The introduction of ultrasound has further modified how these blocks are performed and should be integrated into your answer

a) Midclavicular Brachial Plexus Block

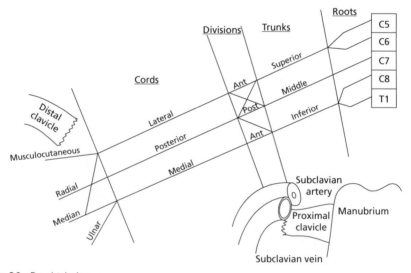

Figure 30. Brachial plexus

- Standard preoperative assessment and procedural consent
  - S   Sterile technique
  - L   Light source
  - I   IV access
  - M Monitoring, NIBP, HR, SpO$_2$
  - R   Resuscitation equipment
  - A   Assistant trained in regional and general anaesthesia
  - G   Ability to administer GA if appropriate
- The jugular notch and ventral acromion are identified, marked, and measured. A line is drawn connecting the two points

- The mid-clavicular approach identifies the midpoint of this line as the puncture site (moved laterally by 0.3cm for every centimetre the clavicle measures <20cm)
- A 50mm nerve-stimulating block needle is inserted vertically and advanced in the sagittal plane from ventral to dorsal
- Care must be taken to avoid medial angulation when advancing the needle as the pleura lies in close proximity (inferomedial direction)
- The cords are usually identified at a depth of 2–3cm. The needle should not be advanced beyond 4cm
- Negative aspiration confirms extravascular placement, followed by chosen LA injection
- Ultrasound infra-clavicular techniques usually focus around the coracoid process as visualization of the needle is easier and the anatomy is easier to identify

b) Cord Identification

i) Posterior Cord
- Wrist or finger extension
- Associated with best results

ii) Medial Cord
- Wrist flexion, thumb adduction
- Accept if surgery is mainly in the ulnar territory
- Often associated with a medial needle position: may need lateral adjustment

iii) Lateral Cord
- Elbow flexion (musculocutaneous)
- Do not accept: too lateral and/or superficial
- Musculocutaneous and axillary nerves leave the plexus sheath before the coracoid process in 50% of patients

iv) Subscapular
- Posterior adduction of the scapula
- Reject block, as outside the plexus sheath

c) Complications

- Pneumothorax
- Intravascular injection
- Intraneural or intrafascicular injection
- Pectoralis haematoma
- Failure

Notes

....
....
....
....
....
....

Reference

Macfarlane A, Anderson K. Infraclavicular brachial plexus blocks. *Continuing Education in Anaesthesia, Critical Care & Pain*, **9**, 139–43, 2009

Q9 Inguinal Region

a) **Outline the nerve supply of structures in the inguinal region (8 marks)**

b) **Describe a regional technique that is adequate to perform a hernia repair under local anaesthesia alone (7 marks)**

c) **List the advantages and complications of this technique (5 marks)**

Aims

The inguinal region is a common area for regional blockade, and presents another anatomy section that should be second nature. This question further explores the candidate's understanding of the nerve supply by examining alternative techniques for blocking the region, and a structured approach is the most thorough. The answer below is one such example of how to tackle this.

a) The Inguinal Region Nerve Supply

  i) Intercostal
- Lateral terminal branches of T11–12 intercostal nerves supply the uppermost regions of this area

  ii) Iliohypogastric
- Branch from L1 anterior primary ramus (occasionally from T12)
- Divides into anterior and lateral branches
  - Lateral branches supply upper gluteal and lateral abdominal wall areas
  - Anterior branches pierce the internal oblique muscle and supply the upper medial aspect of the inguinal region immediately above the external inguinal ring

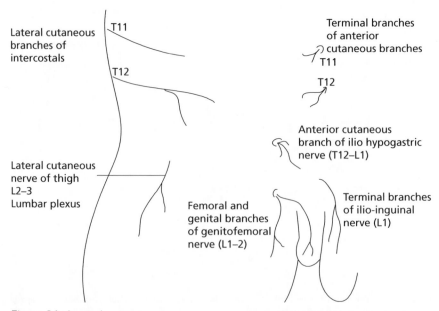

Figure 31. Inguinal region

iii) Ilio-inguinal
- Arises from fusion of T12 and L1 nerve roots and emerges from the lateral border of psoas major
- Provides neural branches to transversus abdominis, internal oblique muscles, and iliohypogastric nerve
- Sensory branches supply pubic symphysis, superior and medial aspect of the femoral triangle, and either the root of the penis and anterior scrotum in males, or the mons pubis and labia majora in females

iv) Genitofemoral
- L1 and L2 ventral primary rami fuse in psoas major to form the nerve trunk
- Divides into genital and femoral branches near the inguinal ligament
  - The genital branch gives motor supply to the cremaster muscle and sensory supply to the spermatic cord, scrotum, and adjacent thigh in males, and cutaneous sensation to the labia majora and adjacent thigh in females
  - The femoral branch supplies sensation to the proximal portion of the femoral triangle

b) Technique

- Standard preoperative assessment and procedural consent
  - S   Sterile equipment
  - L   Light source
  - I   IV access
  - M   Monitoring
  - R   Resuscitation equipment
  - A   Assistant trained in regional and general anaesthesia
  - G   Ability to convert to GA if appropriate
- A blunted needle or block needle is inserted 2cm medial and inferior to the anterior superior iliac spine (ASIS)
- Passage of the needle through the external oblique aponeurosis is confirmed by a click
- Inject 5–8mL of LA after aspirating; minimal resistance should be felt. This will block the ilio-hypogastric branch
- The needle is advanced a further 1–2cm, followed by another click as it crosses the internal oblique. A further 5–8mL of LA will block the ilio-inguinal branch
- Fanwise infiltration around the ASIS will block any neural branches from the ilio-inguinal and hypogastric nerves to improve the efficacy of the block
- The genitofemoral nerve is blocked by a fanwise injection around the pubic tubercle towards the external ring
- Often requires supplementation by the surgeon perioperatively

c) Advantages and Complications

i) Advantages
- Avoids need for GA in patients with severe comorbidities (e.g. COPD)
- Analgesia and anaesthesia is provided
- Earlier readiness for ambulation and discharge home compared with spinal or GA
- Cost-effective
- ↓ postoperative opiate requirement and associated complications

ii) Complications
- Intravascular injection
- Intraperitoneal injection ± bowel or bladder injury
- Failure

- Femoral nerve block
  - May warrant admission overnight
  - Incidence quoted between 1% and 5%

Notes

Q10 Intercostal Nerve

a) **Describe the course of the intercostal nerve (6 marks)**

b) **List the indications for performing an intercostal nerve block (4 marks)**

c) **Describe a technique for performing this block (5 marks)**

d) **List the complications associated with this technique (5 marks)**

Aims

Despite appearing a relatively straightforward topic, it is easy to become caught up on areas of anatomy such as the intercostal nerve, especially as the block is being performed less frequently.

a) Intercostal Nerve

- Ventral and dorsal thoracic spinal nerve roots unite and exit the vertebral canal via the intervertebral foramen, and then divide into the ventral (anterior) and dorsal (posterior) rami
    - The dorsal ramus supplies the extensor muscles of the back and overlying skin
    - The ventral ramus runs in the neurovascular bundle located below the intercostal vein and artery, within the groove on the underside of the corresponding rib, and supplies motor innervation to the intercostal and transverse thoracic muscles

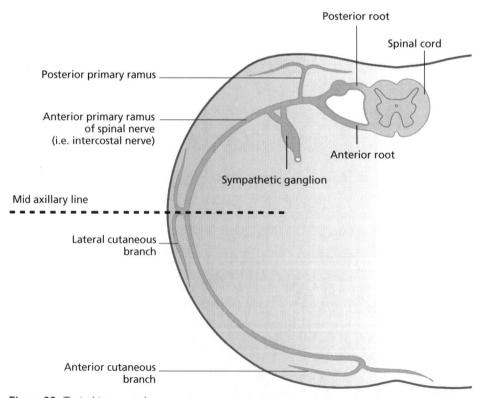

Figure 32. Typical intercostal nerve

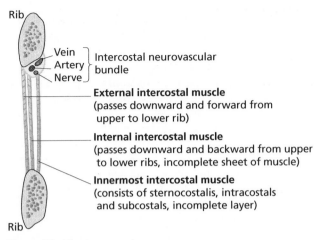

Figure 33. The intercostal space

- Initially lies between the pleura and posterior intercostal membrane, and then moves to lie between the internal and innermost intercostal muscle layers
- Gives off a lateral branch around the mid-axillary line to supply the overlying lateral skin of the corresponding dermatome to the mid-clavicular line
- Terminates as the anterior cutaneous branch, which is a sensory supply from the mid-axillary line to the anterior midline of the chest wall
- Communicating branches cross intercostal spaces, often uniting with the ventral ramus at the origin of the lateral cutaneous branch
- Grey and white rami communicantes connect the intercostal nerve to the sympathetic chain

b) Indications

- Rib fractures
- Intercostal procedures (e.g. intercostal drain insertion)
- Postoperative analgesia for thoracic and upper abdominal surgery
  - ◆ An adjunct technique, generally superseded now by paravertebral, epidural, or TAP blocks
  - ◆ Classically, blockade of two dermatomes above and below the incision
- Acute herpes zoster and neurolysis for chronic pain syndromes (coeliac plexus block is required for visceral analgesia)

c) Technique

- Standard preoperative assessment and procedural consent
  - S   Sterile equipment
  - L   Light source
  - I   IV access
  - M   Monitoring
  - R   Resuscitation equipment
  - A   Assistant trained in regional and general anaesthesia
  - G   Ability to convert to GA if required or appropriate
- An injection is to be made at or before the angle of the rib to block the nerve before it divides
- Tether the skin and palpate the rib to be blocked

- Insert the needle 20° cephalad until the lower border of the rib is encountered
- Release the skin to allow the needle to realign horizontally
- Walk the tip of the needle off the lower border of the rib and advance 2–3mm to puncture the innermost intercostal muscle
- Aspirate and inject 2–5mL of LA solution
- Average depth of pleura from the posterior aspect of the rib is 8mm; therefore advancing beyond 3–5mm greatly ↑ the risk of pneumothorax

d) Complications

i) Due to Needle
- Vessel injury
- Pneumothorax or visceral injury (quoted as <1%)
- Subarachnoid injection: anatomical studies have revealed that the dural cuff can extend as far as 8cm along the ventral root

ii) Due to the Local Anaesthetic
- Respiratory distress in patients with concurrent respiratory disease because of blockade of intercostals or, more commonly, the diaphragm in lower nerve root blocks
- Systemic toxicity due to intravascular injection
- Rich blood supply results in rapid absorption of LA; caution is exercised with multiple-level or continual infusion techniques
- Spread to adjacent levels, including sympathetic chain blockade, has been demonstrated with dye studies

Notes

Q11 Internal Jugular Vein

a) **Describe the course of the internal jugular vein (7 marks)**

b) **Outline the clinical relevance of this vein for anaesthetists in theatre and ICU (6 marks)**

c) **List the complications of cannulation of this vessel (7 marks)**

Aims

An understanding of the relative anatomy and course of the internal jugular vein is considered a core area for anaesthetists who use this vein frequently for venous access. Awareness and familiarity with both image-guided and blind techniques should also be part of your portfolio of common procedures that you are confident to describe.

a) Anatomy of the IJV

- Formed by the unification of the sigmoid sinus and inferior petrosal sinus

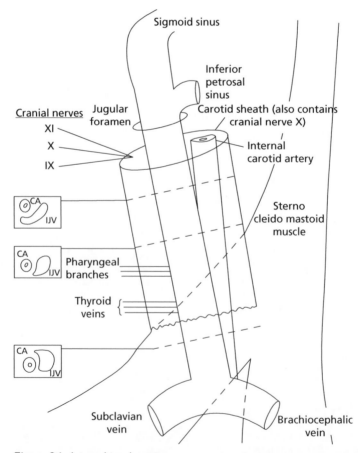

Figure 34. Internal jugular vein

- Exits the skull via the jugular foramen and runs down the neck within the carotid sheath together with the internal carotid artery and the vagus nerve
- The recurrent laryngeal nerve lies medial to this sheath
- The relationship of the artery and vein varies in individuals: the most common pattern is for the vein to lie posteriorly at the base of the skull, lateral to the artery in the mid-neck, moving to lie anterolateral to the artery in the lower half of neck
- The upper half of the vessel is superficial and the lower half lies deep to the sternocleidomastoid muscle
- It terminates by joining with the subclavian vein behind the manubrium sternum to form the brachiocephalic vein

b) Relevance

i) Theatre
- Common site for central access: easy to identify and access
- Placement of central line for measuring CVP
- Placement of multi-lumen catheter for running multiple infusions, i.e. vasopressors, or vaso-irritant solutions such as potassium or amiodarone
- Placement of large-bore line (e.g. pulmonary artery catheter sheath introducer to facilitate rapid fluid resuscitation)
- Access for the introduction of pacing wires
- Cardiac catheter studies

ii) ICU
- Inotrope infusions
- Flow monitoring (e.g. pulse contour continuous cardiac output)
- Total parenteral nutrition
- Jugular venous bulb saturation measurement
- Sedation
- Renal replacement therapy (e.g. haemofiltration)

c) Complications of Cannulation

i) Due to Needle
- Pneumothorax or haemothorax:
  - intrapleural placement of line
- Carotid artery puncture:
  - intimal dissection
  - flow obstruction
  - emboli
- Local haematoma in neck
- Nerve injury (e.g. vagus or recurrent laryngeal nerve)
- Thyroid puncture
- Thoracic duct puncture (commonly, left-sided low approach)

ii) Due to Line
- Arrythmias following line insertion
- Air embolism
- Infection
- Vessel stenosis
- Thrombosis
- Proximal flow obstruction
- Cardiac tamponade following erosion of the vessel wall from the tip of the line
- Subclavian vein cannulation

NICE published guidelines in 2002 suggesting the use of ultrasound for placement of all internal jugular lines to reduce the incidence of misplacement

Notes

Reference

http://www.nice.org.uk/nicemedia/pdf/Ultrasound_49_GUIDANCE.pdf (accessed 2 December 2009)

Q12 Interpleural Block

a) List the indications for performing an interpleural block (6 marks)

b) Describe a known technique for performing this block (8 marks)

c) Outline the complications associated with interpleural blocks (6 marks)

Aims

The interpleural block is a very effective procedure for unilateral mid-trunk analgesia and lends itself to a variety of scenarios. An understanding of the plane of local anaesthetic administration makes prediction of complications easier. There are a variety of techniques for performing the block. One example is given below.

a) Indications

i) Surgical
- Breast procedures: mastectomy, reconstructions, biopsies
- Cardiothoracics: thoracotomy, thoracic sympathectomy, intercostal chest drain insertion
- Abdominal: laparoscopic or open cholecystectomy, renal surgery, extracorporeal shock wave lithotripsy, percutaneous nephrostomy or nephrolithotomy, generalized abdominal surgery (bilateral blocks required), percutaneous hepatic or biliary drainage

ii) Trauma
- Thoracic chest wall trauma, although caution if haemothorax suspected or present
- Multiple rib fractures (catheter insertion and continuous LA infusion is ideal)

iii) Chronic Pain
- Acute herpes zoster and post-herpetic neuralgia
- Chronic regional and ischaemic pain syndromes of upper limb
- Chest wall or organ visceral pain
- Cancer pain (e.g. oesophageal, pancreatic, upper abdominal organs)
- Acute or chronic pancreatitis pain
- Tumour invasion of brachial plexus

b) Interpleural Block Technique

- Standard preoperative assessment and procedural consent
  - S   Sterile equipment
  - L   Light source
  - I   IV access
  - M   Monitoring
  - R   Resuscitation equipment
  - A   Assistant trained in regional and general anaesthesia
  - G   Ability to convert to GA if appropriate
- A 1L bag of crystalloid fluid with a giving set and three-way tap is prepared and primed
- The patient is supine with the block-side arm abducted and the hand placed behind the head. The skin is cleaned and LA is infiltrated if the patient is awake
- A 16G Tuohy needle is inserted at the chosen entry point (usually 4th–8th intercostal space, mid-anterior axillary line) down onto the rib and the stylet is removed. The three-way tap–giving set–saline infusion is attached to the end of the Tuohy needle and the infusion switched on

- The Tuohy needle is 'walked' off the superior border of the rib. At this point there should be virtually no flow through the infusion, at best a few drops. Ventilation should be paused in a paralysed patient, and advancement of the needle must only occur in the expiratory phase of a spontaneously breathing patient
- The needle is advanced slowly until the parietal pleura is punctured; at this point the infusion will run freely. The three-way tap is turned off to the patient and a syringe with chosen LA attached. After negative aspiration, LA is injected; there should be minimal resistance to injection. The needle is then removed with the saline infusion running
- Typically requires a large volume to achieve optimal block, ranging from 20 to 40mL. Caution with toxic LA doses
- An epidural catheter may be inserted to provide a continuous LA infusion or repeated LA boluses

c) Complications

i) Related to Technique
- Pneumothorax
- Intrabronchial injection
- Bronchopleural fistula
- Catheter misplacement
- Infection
- Ipsilateral bronchospasm

ii) Related to LA Injection or Infusion
- Systemic LA toxicity
- Intravascular injection
- Direct myocardial depression
- Horner's syndrome
- Phrenic nerve palsy

Notes

....

....

....

....

....

....

....

References

Dravid RM, Paul RE. Interpleural block: Part 1. *Anaesthesia*, **62**: 1039–49, 2007
Dravid RM, Paul RE. Interpleural block: Part 2. *Anaesthesia*, **62**: 1143–53, 2007
Scott PV. Interpleural regional analgesia: detection of the interpleural space by saline infusion. *British Journal of Anaesthesia*, **66**: 131–3, 1991

Q13 Larynx

a) Describe the surface anatomy of the larynx (5 marks)
b) Outline the important cartilage structures within the larynx (7 marks)
c) Which muscles are involved in vocal cord manipulation? (5 marks)
d) What is the nerve supply to the larynx? (3 marks)

Aims

Although the Final Examination explores clinical applications of basic science knowledge, occasionally a straightforward anatomy question may appear. Further clinical applications in a viva setting could include the consequences of nerve damage.

a) Surface Anatomy of the Larynx

- Boundaries are from the base of the tongue superiorly extending to the cricoid cartilage inferiorly

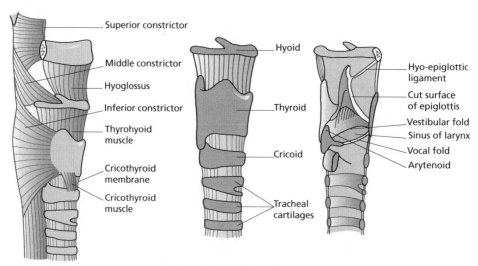

Figure 35. Muscle, cartilage, and sagittal section of the larynx

- Lies opposite C3–6 in adult males; smaller and more cephalad in women and children
- Hyoid bone: a U-shaped bone with two horns posteriorly articulating with the mandible. Lies adjacent to the C3 vertebral body

b) Cartilages

- Six cartilages articulating with each other to form the functional larynx
- i) Epiglottis
  - Large U-shaped structure found at the base of the tongue

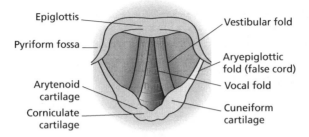

Figure 36. The view at laryngoscopy

ii) Thyroid Cartilage (pair)
- Large square cartilages that join in the midline to form the 'Adam's apple'
- Lies below the hyoid bone, connected by the thyrohyoid membrane, which is pierced by the superior laryngeal vessels and the internal branch of the superior laryngeal nerve
- Articulates with the cricoid cartilage inferiorly via the cricothyroid membrane

iii) Cricoid Cartilage
- Complete cartilage ring, wider posteriorly
- Articulates with the thyroid and arytenoid cartilages

iv) Arytenoid Cartilage
- Pyramid-shaped pair of cartilages
- Smooth base articulates with the cricoid cartilage
- Anterior process attaches to the vocal folds
- Posterior muscular process
- Apex articulates with corniculate cartilages

v) Corniculate Cartilage
- Pair of cartilages that lie at the apex of the arytenoids, forming tubercles in the posterior aryepiglottic folds

vi) Cuneiform Cartilage
- Pair of cartilages that lie in front of the corniculate cartilages

c) Muscles

i) Extrinsic Muscles
- Responsible for anchoring the larynx to the adjacent structures in the head and neck:
  - sternothyroid
  - thyrohyoid
  - inferior pharyngeal constrictors

ii) Intrinsic Muscles
- Responsible for manipulation of the vocal folds for phonation or coughing
- Abduction (i.e. cords apart)
  - Posterior cricoarytenoid
- Adduction (i.e. cords towards midline)
  - Lateral cricoarytenoids and unpaired inter-arytenoid muscles

- Cord tensors
  - Cricothyroid (the only intrinsic muscle outside the larynx and the only muscle supplied by the external branch of the superior laryngeal nerve)
- Cord relaxors
  - Thyroarytenoid muscles
  - Vocalis

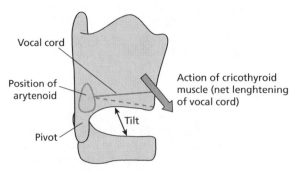

Figure 37. Extrinsic muscles of the larynx

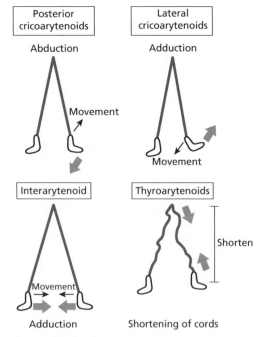

Figure 38. Cord movements

d) Nerve supply

- Vagus nerve divides into the superior and recurrent laryngeal nerves
- i) Superior laryngeal nerve
    - Internal laryngeal nerve: supplies the inferior epiglottis and sensation above the vocal cords
    - External laryngeal nerve: supplies motor to cricothyroid muscle
- ii) Recurrent laryngeal nerve:
    - Sensation below the vocal cords
    - Motor to all remaining intrinsic muscles of the larynx

Notes

Q14 Nerve Supply of the Hand

a) **Describe the sensory nerve supply of the hand (10 marks)**

b) **Describe techniques for blocking the ulnar, median, and radial nerves at the elbow and wrist (10 marks)**

Aims

Knowledge of the distal upper limb blocks is vital as it allows us to supplement 'missed' nerve roots during more proximal brachial plexus blockade.

a) Sensory Nerve Supply of Hand (Four Nerves)

i) Ulnar
- C8–T1 nerve roots, medial cord of brachial plexus
- Dorsal and palmar cutaneous branches arise above the wrist
- Palmar branch: supplies medial aspect of palm over hypothenar eminence
- Dorsal branch: supplies dorsal ulnar border of the hand; at the wrist it lies lateral to the flexor carpi ulnaris tendon

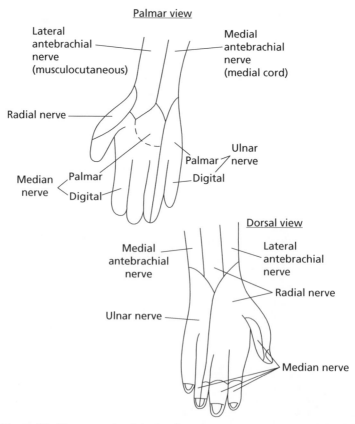

Figure 39. Nerve supply of the hand

- In the hand, the nerve divides into superficial and deep terminal branches
  - Superficial branch is sensory: supplies ulnar 1½ fingers
  - Deep branch is motor

ii) Median
- C6–T1 nerve roots; medial and lateral roots of the median nerve from medial and lateral cords of the brachial plexus
- Palmar cutaneous nerve arises several centimetres above the wrist and supplies the radial side of the palm
- Nerve lies under the palmaris longus tendon at the wrist and ends just distal to the flexor retinaculum
- Palmar digital nerves give sensory branches to the radial 3½ fingers and the thenar eminence

iii) Radial
- C5–T1 nerve roots; posterior cord of the brachial plexus
- Nerve passes deep to the tendon of brachioradialis to reach the dorsum of the hand, crossing superficially to the tendons of the anatomical snuffbox
- Divides into multiple digital branches to supply the dorsal thumb base, the radial side of the back of hand, and the back of the radial 3½ fingers

iv) Musculocutaneous
- C5–7 root values; continuation of the lateral cord of the brachial plexus
- Terminal branch is the lateral antebrachial cutaneous nerve
- Divides into posterior and anterior branches to supply skin along the radial forearm and wrist

b) Nerve Blocks

Ultrasound use is becoming more popular for these distal blocks
- Standard preoperative assessment and procedural consent
  - S   Sterile equipment
  - L   Light source
  - I   IV access
  - M   Monitoring
  - R   Resuscitation equipment
  - A   Assistant trained in regional and general anaesthesia
  - G   Ability to convert to GA if appropriate

i) Elbow
   Ulnar
   - A LA injection is made proximal to the fibrous tunnel at the medial epicondyle
   - Avoid injections in the sulcus as the tight fibrous sheath is thought to be associated with a high incidence of post-block neural damage

   Median
   - The median nerve is found by directing an appropriate needle immediately medial to the brachial pulse in the antecubital fossa

   Radial
   - Palpate the groove between the lateral border of the biceps and brachioradialis muscles. Injection point is 1–2cm proximal to the elbow crease, aiming for the lateral epicondyle

ii) Wrist
   Ulnar
   - Approach from the ulnar border to reduce the risk of arterial puncture

- Identify the medial border of the flexi carpi ulnaris tendon and inject LA 2cm proximal to the wrist crease
- May miss dorsal and palmar branches given off earlier in the forearm

Median
- Advance a needle 2–4cm proximal to wrist crease between the flexi carpi radialis and palmaris longus tendons and inject LA

Radial
- Terminal branches are blocked with a ring block directed around the radial border of the wrist
- LA is injected at the tip of the radial styloid with a further injection around the surrounding area to cover the branches of this nerve

Notes

Q15 Paravertebral Space

You wish to perform paravertebral blocks for a 53-year-old woman listed for a right mastectomy.

a) Outline the borders and contents of the paravertebral space (6 marks)

b) Describe the technique for blocking nerves in this area (6 marks)

c) List the indications (4 marks) and complications (4 marks) of this technique

Aims

Although you may not have performed this block, it is possible to give a good account if you have a clear idea of the boundaries of the paravertebral space. Having already appeared in the written final examination, it may also crop up in the oral examination.

a) Paravertebral Space Anatomy

- The name given to the potential space found on each side lateral to the bony vertebral column in the thoracolumbar region

i) Boundaries
  - Anterolateral: parietal pleura in thorax, and sacrospinalis and psoas muscle in abdomen
  - Medial: pedicals and posterolateral aspect of the vertebral body and intervertebral foramina

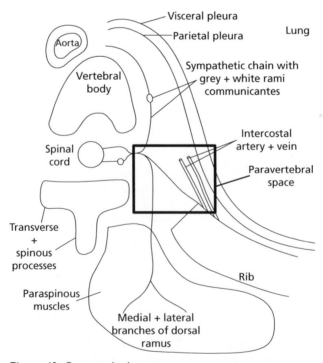

Figure 40. Paravertebral space

- Posterior: transverse process and costo-transverse ligament in thorax
- Superior: head of adjacent rib in thoracic region

ii) Contents
- Spinal nerve roots emerging from the intervertebral foramina enter this space before giving off white rami communicantes to join with the sympathetic chain. The nerve root divides into dorsal and ventral branches before leaving this space
- Sympathetic chain
- Fat
- Lymph nodes
- Vessels

b) Paravertebral Nerve Block

- Standard preoperative assessment and procedural consent
  - S   Sterile equipment
  - L   Light source
  - I   IV access
  - M   Monitoring
  - R   Resuscitation equipment
  - A   Assistant trained in regional and general anaesthesia
  - G   Ability to convert to GA if appropriate
- Technique can be either single-shot or at multiple levels; a catheter may be inserted for continued analgesia
- Position is either sitting or lateral
- Key landmark to identify is the spinous process at the level to be blocked. A mark is placed 2.5cm laterally, correlating with the transverse process of the vertebral body for the lumbar region, or the vertebral body below for the thoracic region owing to the sloping nature of thoracic transverse processes
- An appropriate needle (blunt/atraumatic tip or Tuohy) is inserted perpendicular to all planes to a depth of 3–5cm and bony contact is made with the transverse process
- The needle is walked off the transverse process caudally and advanced a further 1cm (a subtle pop may be felt in the thoracic region as the costo-transverse ligament is crossed)
- Following negative aspiration, 3–5ml of LA is injected per level
- Alternatively, a catheter may be advanced and LA infusion commenced

c) Indications and Complications

i) Indications
- Analgesia for:
  - breast surgery
  - thoracic surgery
  - open cholecystectomy
  - nephrectomy
  - hernia repair
  - video-assisted thoracoscopy
- Trauma (e.g. fractured ribs)
- Symptom control of hyperhydrosis
- Chronic pain conditions e.g. post-herpetic neuralgia, complex regional pain syndrome, malignancy

ii) Complications
- Inadvertent intravascular injection
- Local anaesthetic toxicity

- Pneumothorax
- Extradural or intrathecal spread via intervertebral foramina
- Ipsilateral Horner's syndrome
- Haematoma
- Infection
- Nerve injury
- Bilateral injections: hypotension following sympathetic block

Notes

Reference

Tighe SQM, Greene MD, Rajadurai N. Paravertebral block. *Continuing Education in Anaesthesia, Critical Care & Pain*, **10**, 133–7, 2010

Q16 Popliteal Fossa Block

a) Describe the region supplied by nerves arising from the popliteal fossa (8 marks)
b) What motor responses would you get upon stimulating these nerves? (3 marks)
c) Outline a technique for performing this block (9 marks)

Aims

This question examines your knowledge of a peripheral nerve that you may not have blocked before, but by understanding its innervation you can predict when it is likely to be used clinically. The emphasis of the question is describing the sensory and motor innervation, and to answer all stems of the question answers in list style with a clear structure are required for the other sections

a) Popliteal Fossa Nerves and Their Cutaneous Distribution

- i) Tibial (Medial)
    - Main terminal branch of sciatic nerve
    - Sensory branches
        - Sural nerve arises in popliteal fossa:
            - supplies the lateral border of the foot
        - Medial plantar nerve (arises at the level of the flexor retinaculum):
            - supplies the medial two-thirds of the sole of the foot and the plantar medial 3½ toes
        - Lateral plantar nerve (also arises at the level of the flexor retinaculum):
            - supplies the lateral third of the sole of the foot and the plantar lateral 1½ toes
- ii) Peroneal (Lateral)
    - Common peroneal nerve branches from the sciatic nerve at a variable distance above the popliteal fossa
    - Divides into deep and superficial peroneal nerves
    - Sensory branches
        - Sural communicating nerve is absent in 20% cases:
            - joins with the sural nerve from the popliteal fossa
        - Superficial peroneal nerve:
            - lower outer aspect of the lower leg
            - terminal branches innervate the dorsum of the foot
        - Deep peroneal nerve: first web space

b) Responses Elicited Upon Stimulation of These Nerves

- Tibial: plantar flexion of toes and inversion of foot
- Common peroneal: dorsiflexion of toes and eversion of the foot
- Sciatic: combination of the above
- Isolated twitches of the calf muscle are likely to be due to stimulation of direct sciatic branches to the gastrocnemius muscle and do not signify correct needle-tip placement

c) Technique

- Standard preoperative assessment and procedural consent
    - S Sterile equipment
    - L Light source
    - I IV access

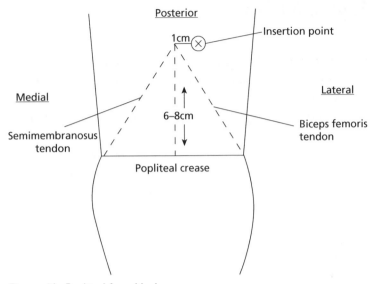

Figure 41. Popliteal fossa block

M   Monitoring
R   Resuscitation equipment
A   Assistant trained in regional and general anaesthesia
G   Ability to convert to GA if appropriate
- If awake, the patient is positioned prone and asked to flex and extend his/her knee to aid identification of the mid-popliteal skin crease
- If asleep, the patient may be supine with the leg straight-raised by an assistant, or transferred to the lateral decubitus position
- Palpate the tendons of the biceps femoris (lateral) and semitendinosus and semimembranosus (medial)
- Locate the inter-tendinous gap and mark a site, usually 6–8cm proximal to the mid-popliteal skin crease
- The needle is introduced perpendicular to the skin and advanced until foot stimulation is obtained
- Failure to identify a twitch usually indicates a more lateral position of the nerve trunk; direct the needle laterally after withdrawal to just under the skin, or alternatively try a puncture site 1cm lateral to the original site
- After negative aspiration slowly inject LA

Notes

....

....

....

....

....

....

Q17 Sciatic Nerve

a) **Outline the course of the sciatic nerve (6 marks)**

b) **Describe how you would block the sciatic nerve using the anterior (Beck) approach (9 marks)**

c) **List the potential complications of sciatic nerve blockade (5 marks)**

Aims

As demonstrated in a recent SAQ paper, understanding the different approaches to the sciatic nerve should be within your repertoire of answers even if you have not performed some of the less common techniques.

a) The Sciatic Nerve

- The largest peripheral nerve in the body formed from the anterior primary rami of L4–S3. Main branch of the sacral plexus
- The nerve roots converge on the anterior surface of the piriformis muscle before exiting via the inferior portion of the greater sciatic foramen as the sciatic nerve
- It leaves the pelvis and enters the thigh by passing midway between the ischial tuberosity and the greater trochanter
- It descends in the posterior compartment of the thigh towards the popliteal fossa
- The nerve divides to form its two main terminal branches, the tibial and common peroneal nerves, approximately 6–10cm above the popliteal fossa, although it is possible for the two branches to divide more proximally
- The nerve trunk is composed of two nerves bound together in one epineurium. The common peroneal nerve usually lies lateral to the tibial medial

b) Sciatic Nerve Block

- Standard preoperative assessment and procedural consent
  - S   Sterile equipment
  - L   Light source
  - I   IV access
  - M   Monitoring
  - R   Resuscitation equipment
  - A   Assistant trained in regional and general anaesthesia
  - G   Ability to convert to GA if appropriate

i) Anterior (Beck or Meier) Approach
  - Patient lies supine
  - Line 1 extends from the anterior superior iliac spine to the pubic tubercle
  - Line 2 is parallel to line 1, beginning at the greater trochanter and extending to the medial border of the thigh
  - At the junction of the medial and middle thirds, connect the two lines perpendicularly
  - The puncture site is where this perpendicular crosses line 2
  - A 150mm needle is advanced posteriorly to touch the femur, withdrawn, and angled to pass under the medial border of the femur, usually 2–3cm further (average depth 10–13cm)
  - Femoral nerve stimulation is not uncommon initially; if performing in an awake patient, perform a femoral block first

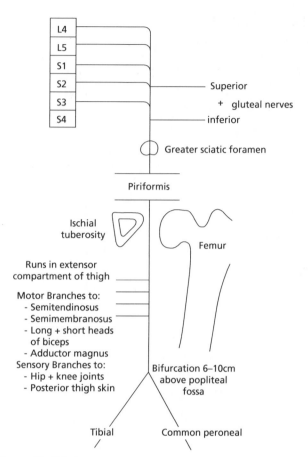

Figure 42. Sciatic nerve

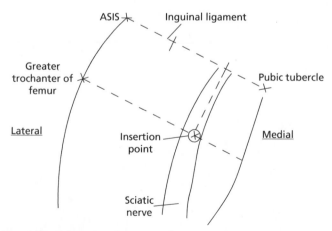

Figure 43. Anterior sciatic nerve block

c) Complications

i) Due to Needle
- Mechanical trauma to the nerve (e.g. needle trauma, intraneuronal (intrafascicular) injection)
- Inadvertent needle placement into unwanted locations and subsequent injury, i.e. haematoma formation
- Vessel injury

ii) Due to Local Anaesthetic
- Systemic toxicity due to intravascular injection
- Neuronal ischaemia due to pressure induced by local anaesthetic
- Neurotoxicity of local anaesthetics, especially when using large volumes of local anaesthetic
- Drug error (injection of wrong drug type, volume, concentration)
- Infection
- Failure of the desired effect of the block
- Specific concerns with sciatic nerve blocks include avoidance of adrenaline-containing solutions as the blood supply to the nerve is easily compromised.

Notes

Q18 Spinal Cord

a) **Describe the arterial blood supply to the spinal cord (13 marks)**
b) **Discuss the consequences of interruption of the anterior spinal artery (7 marks)**

Aims

Although initially appearing complex, the blood supply of the cord is easier when broken down. Understanding the territorial nature of the arterial perfusion makes it easier to recall the clinical patterns seen following interruption to these vessels and their management. An understanding of the venous drainage is also necessary as this could easily be linked to questions regarding epidural procedures

a) Blood Supply

- Two posterior spinal arteries
  - Arise from the posterior inferior cerebellar artery and vertebral arteries and descend to lie medial to the roots of the posterior cervical nerve
  - Supply posterior third of spinal cord fasciculus gracilis/cuneatus (vibration, light touch, proprioception)
  - Significant variation exists in this branching
  - There are often excellent collateral anastomoses
- One anterior spinal artery
  - Midline vessel that begins at the foramen magnum by union of anterior spinal branches of the vertebral artery (on the rostral surface of the medulla between pyramids)
  - Descends in the midline fissure, producing several branches to supply the anterior two-thirds of the spinal cord
- Supplemental branches: 25–40 additional vessels join from adjacent arteries as the spinal cord descends in the vertebral column:
  - Cervical/upper thoracic supply: vertebral, thyrocostal, subclavian, and costocervical arteries

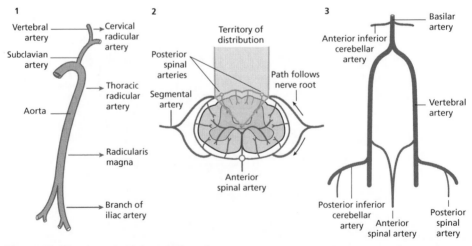

Figure 44. Blood supply of the spinal cord

- ◆ T4–T9 intercostals (anterior and posterior branches)
- ◆ Below T9, the main feeder vessel is the radicularis magna, or artery of Adamkiewicz. In 80% of patients, this vessel enters the cord via the intervertebral foramina on the left side of the patient, being derived from the abdominal aorta (commonly around T10–T11)
- ◆ In around 15% of patients, the radicularis magna arises at T5 level, resulting in the lower cord receiving a greater proportion of its blood supply from the iliac vessels, and a resultant higher incidence of cauda equina syndrome if these vessels are interrupted
- ◆ Lumbar supply: iliac, lumbar, and lateral sacral arteries
- • Functional blood supply
  - ◆ Divided into three broad zones with good horizontal cross-over
  - ◆ Poor vertical overlap renders the cord vulnerable to watershed ischaemic insults

b) Interruption of the Anterior Spinal Artery

- • The main implications for this vessel are focused around ruptured abdominal aortic aneurysms (AAAs)
- • Hypotension, worsened in the presence of atherosclerosis and luminal narrowing, can render a large section of the thoracolumbar cord ischaemic and potentially infarcted
- • This endpoint may also be seen during both elective and emergency open AAA repair as the vessel is lost during graft interposition
- • The vessel is also at risk of embolic occlusion
- • Associated clinical signs include the following
  - ◆ Loss of motor function below the level of the lesion (corticospinal and vestibulospinal)
  - ◆ Loss of temperature and pain perception below the level of the lesion (spinothalamic)
  - ◆ Preserved dorsal columns mean that vibration, proprioception, and light touch remain unaltered

Notes

Q19 Stellate Ganglion

a) What are the indications for stellate ganglion blockade? (6 marks)

b) Describe a technique for blocking this structure (7 marks)

c) List the complications of this block (7 marks)

Aims

Although rare, and often not witnessed by the majority of trainees, this block remains a popular examination theme. The key is understanding its adjacent features, as side effects and complications are a common feature in questions around this topic.

a) Indications

i) Sympathetic-Mediated Pain
   * Complex Regional Pain Syndrome type I and type II
   * Refractory angina
   * Phantom limb pain
   * Herpes zoster
   * Shoulder or hand syndrome
   * Angina

ii) Vascular Insufficiency
   * Raynaud's syndrome
   * Scleroderma
   * Frostbite
   * Obliterative vascular disease
   * Vasospasm
   * Trauma
   * Emboli

b) Blockade Technique

* Standard preoperative assessment and procedural consent
  S Sterile technique
  L Light source
  I IV access
  M Monitoring: BP, HR SpO$_2$
  R Resuscitation equipment
  A Assistant trained in regional and general anaesthesia
  G Ability to administer GA if appropriate

i) Anterior Approach
   * Patient supine with head extended; some advocate turning the head to the contra-lateral side and opening the mouth
   * At the level of C6 (cricoid cartilage), displace the carotid sheath laterally whilst the trachea is moved medially
   * Insert a 25mm 25G needle directly perpendicular to the skin onto the transverse process of C6 (Chassaignac's tubercle)
   * Withdraw the needle approximately 5 mm and then inject approximately 20mL of LA solution

- A large volume is required for cephalic and caudal migration to block the lower thoracic segments joining the ganglion
- Requires fluoroscopic confirmation of needle position before injection of LA

d) Complications

i) Misplaced Needle
   - Haematoma from vascular trauma (carotid, IJV, vertebral); possibility of airway compression if large
   - Nerve trunk injury (vagus and recurrent laryngeal nerve)
   - Brachial plexus root injury
   - Pneumothorax
   - Haemothorax
   - Chylothorax (thoracic duct injury)
   - Oesophageal perforation

ii) Spread of Local Anaesthetic
   - Intravascular injection:
   - Carotid artery
   - Vertebral artery
   - Internal jugular vein
   - Neuraxial or brachial plexus spread: epidural or intrathecal block
   - Brachial plexus anaesthesia or injury (intraneural injection)
   - Local spread: hoarseness (recurrent laryngeal nerve), elevated hemidiaphragm (phrenic nerve)
   - Horner's syndrome (ptosis, meiosis, enopthalmos)

iii) Infection
   - Soft tissue (abscess)
   - Neuraxial (meningitis)
   - Osteitis

Notes

Q20 Sub-Tenon's Eye Block

a) **List the advantages and disadvantages of regional anaesthesia for ophthalmic surgery (6 marks)**

b) **Describe a recognized technique for performing a sub-Tenon's block (9 marks)**

c) **List the complications of the sub-Tenon's block (5 marks)**

Aims

Beginning with a broad question regarding indications and contraindications for ophthalmic blocks, this question then moves on to the description of the sub-Tenon's block, which offers both anaesthesia and akinesia. You should be well versed in the anatomy around the globe in general, but this block in particular has probably become the primary form of regional ocular anaesthesia. You should be able to justify why.

a) Regional Anaesthesia for Ophthalmic Surgery

   i) Advantages
   - More suitable for day-case surgery
   - Avoids complications of GA (e.g. multiple comorbidities, PONV, sore throat)
   - Postoperative analgesia
   - Potential faster turnover of list
   - Provides both analgesia and akinesia
   - Blunting of occulo-cardiac reflex

   ii) Disadvantages
   - Chronic cough is poorly tolerated
   - Patient unable to lie flat (e.g. back pain, heart failure, shortness of breath)
   - Anticoagulation: INR >2.5
   - Previous retinal detachment contraindicated
   - Trauma to eye
   - Local infection
   - Poor for long surgery

b) Sub-Tenon's Block

- Ideal eye block as it provides optimal surgical conditions (anaesthesia and akinesia) without risk of retro- and peribulbar techniques
- Standard preoperative assessment and procedural consent
   S   Sterile equipment
   L   Light source
   I   IV access
   M   Monitoring
   R   Resuscitation equipment
   A   Assistant trained in regional and general anaesthesia
   G   Ability to convert to GA if appropriate
- Technique aims to dissect down to Tenon's capsule, a fascial layer of connective tissue that surrounds both the globe and the extra-ocular muscles.
- The axial length is checked preoperatively: a length >26mm carries an increased risk of globe perforation

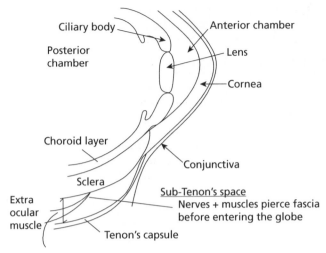

Figure 45. Sub-Tenon's anatomy

- Conjunctival block with topical LA eye drops (e.g. proxymetacaine); iodine drops are also inserted
  - An eyelid retractor is inserted and the patient is asked to look upwards and outwards
  - Locate the inferonasal quadrant and lift a small tent of conjunctiva with forceps at the midpoint between the medial limbus and medial canthus
  - Make a small incision through the conjunctiva with a pair of ophthalmic scissors
  - Blunt dissect down through Tenon's fascia to the sclera
  - A blunt Tenon's 19G cannula is inserted with its tip against the sclera, as it is navigated posteriorly with minimal resistance
  - Resistance due to incorrect tissue plane dissection is solved with redirection of the cannula
  - Occasionally the needle may encounter a fibrous band at the equator, correlating with insertion of the extra-ocular muscles; gentle pressure will overcome this
  - Aspirate and inject LA
  - Mild proptosis of the globe confirms correct spread of the block
  - Some anterior spread of the LA solution is normal; however, excessive chemosis suggests subconjunctival spread, providing analgesia but not akinesia
  - Remove the cannula and gently massage the globe to aid retrograde spread of LA solution; some surgeons prefer a pressure device

c) Complications of the Block

i) Related to the Needle
  - Relatively low because of use of blunt needle
  - Dural puncture and subarachnoid injection
  - Vascular injury and retrobulbar haemorrhage (avoid superior medial quadrant)
  - Scleral perforation
  - Subconjunctival haemorrhage and chemosis
  - Muscle injury

ii) Related to the Local Anaesthetic
   • Subarachnoid injection and spread of LA
   • Intravascular injection
   • Anaphylaxis
   • Diplopia
   • Raised IOP

Notes

Q21 **TAP Block**

a) Describe i) a blind technique and ii) an ultrasound-guided technique for performing a transversus abdominis plexus (TAP) block (11 marks)

b) List the indications and limitations of this technique (9 marks)

Aims

A relatively new block increasingly being used in a variety of surgical procedures, the TAP block is current and therefore likely to crop up in the examination somewhere. A good core understanding of the innervation of the abdominal wall acts as a basis for how this block works.

a) Techniques

- Standard preoperative assessment and procedural consent
    - S Sterile equipment and technique
    - L Light source
    - I IV access
    - M Monitoring
    - R Resuscitation equipment
    - A Assistant trained in regional and general anaesthesia
    - G Ability to convert to GA if appropriate
- i) Blind Technique
    - Usually performed in a supine anaesthetised patient
    - Lumbar triangle of Petit identified in the mid-axillary line
        - Base: iliac crest
        - Anterior wall: external oblique muscle
        - Posterior wall: latissimus dorsi
    - Puncture point just behind the mid-axillary line above the iliac crest
    - An appropriately blunted needle is advanced through the skin, and two distinct 'pops' are felt as the needle crosses the fascial planes of the internal oblique and then the transversus abdominis muscles
    - Negative aspiration excludes intravascular placement and LA is slowly injected, periodically aspirating, with minimal resistance

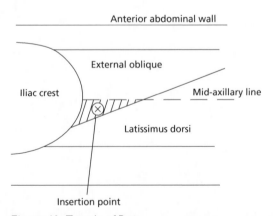

Figure 46. Triangle of Petit

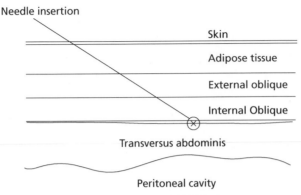

Figure 47. Ultrasound schematic of TAP block

ii) Ultrasound Technique
- A linear array 6–13MHz probe is placed in a horizontal plane between the costal margin and the iliac crest
- An 'in-plane' technique is used to introduce a blunt needle approximately 3–4cm lateral to the probe and advanced so that its tip lies between the internal oblique and transversus abdominis muscle layers
- Negative aspiration confirms extravascular placement
- Spread of LA solution is confirmed as the solution is injected
- Ultrasound allows the discrimination of intramuscular and intrafascial injections

b) Indications
- Reliable spread of LA solution from T10–L1 has been confirmed in both imaging and cadaveric studies, providing good analgesia in lower abdominal operations including the following:

i) Unilateral
- Open appendicectomy
- Open hernia repair

ii) Bilateral
- Laparascopic port incisions
- Pfannenstiel incision (e.g. Caesarean section)
- Abdominal surgery with contraindication to central neuraxial blockade
- Literature reports use in other surgeries (e.g. retropubic prostatectomy) with significant reductions in morphine usage postoperatively
- Subcostal TAP blocks
  - Higher block performed just below costal margin
  - Some studies suggest significant benefit in upper GI surgery, i.e. cholecystectomy

Limitations
- Generally considered to be a safe area for performing regional blockade.
- Needle trauma to local structures, including nerves, blood vessels, and underlying bowel
- A case report of liver injury in patients with undiagnosed hepatomegaly exists
- Intravascular injection
- Infection

- Failure
- Proximal spread of LA solution is difficult to predict above the level of L1
- Often performed as single-shot technique (although catheter techniques are gaining popularity, allowing continued postoperative analgesia)

Notes

Q22 Thoracic Vertebrae

a) **List the joints located between two adjacent thoracic vertebrae (4 marks)**

b) **Describe their nerve supply (6 marks)**

c) **Describe the ligaments found attaching two adjacent lumbar vertebrae (10 marks)**

a) Joints Between Two Adjacent Thoracic Vertebrae

- Cartilaginous joint between bodies (intevertebral disc)
- Synovial joint
  - Zygapophyseal joint (facet joint): superior and inferior facets
  - Costovertebral joint: head of the rib articulates with the body of its own vertebra and the vertebra above
  - Costotransverse joint: angle of upper 10 ribs articulates with transverse process

b) Nerve Supply of the Joints

i) Intervertebral Joint
  - Point of contention.
  - Originally thought to have no innervation, but anatomical studies have described dense innervation of the outer third of the annulus
  - Simple and complex nociceptors have been found
  - Two main sources
    - Anterior plexus:
      - formed by the lumbar sympathetic chain and receives branches from grey rami communicantes
      - supplies the anterior longitudinal ligament

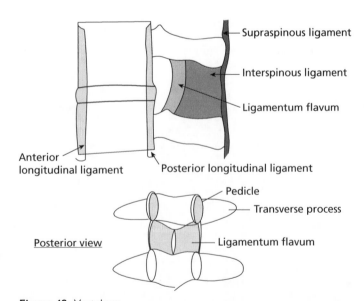

Figure 48. Vertebrae

- ◆ Posterior plexus:
  - ▪ unification of lumbar sinuvertebral nerves
  - ▪ also supplies posterior longitudinal ligament, adjacent dura, and nerve root cuffs
ii) Facet Joint
  - • Medial branch of the dorsal ramus from adjacent spinal nerve
iii) Costovertebral and Costotransverse Joints
  - • Branch from ventral ramus of the corresponding spinal nerve

c) Ligaments Between Two Adjacent Vertebrae

- Anterior longitudinal ligament:
  - ◆ from C1 to the sacrum
  - ◆ attaches to anterior aspect of vertebral bodies
- Posterior longitudinal ligament:
  - ◆ from C2 to the sacrum
  - ◆ attaches to posterior aspect of vertebral bodies and discs
- Ligamenta flava:
  - ◆ collection of short elastic fibres connecting adjacent laminae from axis to first sacral segment
  - ◆ literally means yellow ligament because of its high elastin component
- Interspinous ligament:
  - ◆ connects adjacent spinous process
  - ◆ runs from root to apex of each process
- Supraspinous ligaments:
  - ◆ strong fibrous cord connecting apices of spinous process from C7 to the sacrum
- Ligamentum nuchae:
  - ◆ continuation of the supraspinous ligament above C7
  - ◆ attaches to the external occipital protuberance and median nuchal line
- Intertransverse ligaments:
  - ◆ interposed between the transverse processes
  - ◆ small in the cervical and lumbar regions, but larger and more definite in the thoracic segments
- Intervertebral ligaments:
  - ◆ intervertebral discs are adherent to thin layers of hyaline cartilage covering the ends of the vertebral bodies
  - ◆ in the cervical region these are often replaced with small synovial joints

Notes

....

....

....

....

....

....

Part 4 **Pain Medicine and Analgesia**

Q1 **Addiction**

a) Define tolerance (2 marks), dependence (2 marks), and addiction (3 marks)

b) What principles govern the perioperative analgesic management of a patient with a history of substance abuse? (13 marks)

Aims

We all encounter patients with substance abuse in our regular clinical practice, and they can be extremely challenging both medically and personally. Understanding 'baseline' opioid requirements is the key to successful analgesic management.

a) Definitions

i) Tolerance
  - A pharmacological state where exposure to a drug produces ever-decreasing effects, i.e. continually higher levels of the drug are required to produce an adequate effect

ii) Dependence
  - A physical adaptation where continued use of a substance is necessary to prevent withdrawal symptoms. Often manifested by a drug-class-specific withdrawal syndrome produced by drug cessation or dose reduction

iii) Addiction
  - A spectrum of substance misuse leading to continued abuse despite the actual and potential harm rendered
  - Various factors are involved, including the placing of increasing importance on the substance and the effect it produces, the loss of control over its use, the presence of mood swings, and the potential for relapse states

b) Perioperative Analgesic Management

i) Preoperative
  - Full history (including psychiatric) to elicit current and past substance misuse. Include current medication history to aid safe prescribing, i.e. to avoid potential drug interactions
  - Identify contributing social factors (e.g. alcohol, tobacco, recreational drug use, family circumstances)
  - Clinical examination to recognize signs and symptoms relating to addiction/withdrawal. Initiation and continuation of treatment for withdrawal may affect timing of surgery
  - Frank discussion with patient regarding acceptable behaviour, therapeutic goals, and rationale behind treatment modalities. Aim to gain the trust of the patient
  - Staff to be aware that regular daily intake of opioids may ↑ patient's perception of pain
  - Prescription of appropriate analgesic regimen: avoid 'opioid debt'
    - Use of simple analgesics as adjuncts (e.g. paracetamol, NSAIDs)
    - Controlled regular distribution of sustained-release opioids preferred to the 'peaks and troughs' of short-acting opioids
    - 'Opioid rotation' if current therapy inadequate
    - Consider transdermal opioid patches (e.g. fentanyl)
    - Contact the local drug advisory service and, if advised, replace with methadone regimen on admission.
    - Back-up short-acting opioids for break-through pain

- Prescription to treat potential withdrawal symptoms or complications
- Adequate treatment of anxiety disorders where appropriate
- Ward to be aware of history of substance abuse and potential for drug-seeking behaviour

ii) Intraoperative
- May require premedication with opioids or benzodiazepines
- Polymodal analgesic regimen, i.e. simple analgesia + opioids
- Use regional anaesthesia as the sole technique where possible, including the use of long-acting local anaesthetics
- Consider adjuncts (e.g. magnesium, clonidine, ketamine)

iii) Postoperative
- Do not underestimate analgesic requirements; supplementary opioid doses at supra-normal levels may be required because of tolerance. PCA regimens may have to be altered (e.g. use of background infusion, increased bolus dose size)
- Communicate with the acute pain services. Regular postoperative review and medication adjustments according to progression

Notes

Reference

British Pain Society. *Pain and Substance Misuse: Improving the Patient Experience*. London: British Pain Society, 2007

Q2 Chronic Post-Surgical Pain

a) **What is the definition of chronic post-surgical pain (CPSP)? (2 marks)**

b) **Outline risk factors associated with CPSP (8 marks)**

c) **Describe how anaesthetists may reduce the incidence of CPSP (10 marks)**

Aims

Clinicians are becoming more aware of the phenomenon known as CPSP as a result of long-term follow-up studies. Further discoveries will be made in this field, but there are anaesthetic factors which may affect the development of chronic pain.

a) Definition

- New pain developing after a surgical procedure and lasting for at least two consecutive months with other explanations excluded (i.e. malignancy, infection)
- Cannot be a pre-existing pain

b) Risk Factors

i) Preoperative
- Preoperative pain of any nature: worse if severe or chronic
- Younger age group
- Genetic predisposition resulting in less efficient endogenous modulation of pain signals and central processing
- Anxiety or fear of surgery
- Enhanced preoperative pain sensitivity

ii) Intraoperative
- Long complex surgery
- Nature of surgery: amputation, sternotomy, inguinal hernia repair, and thoracotomy are common triggers
- Previously thought to be related to nerve injury during surgery although this does not appear to be a consistent feature
- Open vs. closed procedures
- Repeat surgery, especially if performed within a year of original surgery

iii) Postoperative
- Severity of postoperative pain is a significant indicator for development of CPSP
- Poor response to analgesic regimen provided postoperatively

c) Techniques to reduce the severity and incidence of CPSP

i) Preoperative
- Identification of high-risk surgery and patients
- Pre-emptive regional analgesia alone is shown to be of little benefit
- Guided imagery therapy has been shown to be of some benefit in decreasing the severity, duration, and incidence of postoperative pain by modulating psychosocial factors related to pain perception

ii) Intraoperative
  - Regional anaesthesia commenced perioperatively and continued afterwards has been shown to significantly reduce the incidence of CPSP
  - Gabapentin administration perioperatively has no effect on incidence in amputation patients. However, when gabapentin was combined with LA in breast surgery, CPSP incidence fell
  - IV ketamine infusions have been used with variable success
  - Clonidine added to RA mixtures has been shown to prolong the duration of block and decrease postoperative pain and CPSP incidence
  - Limited data suggest that multimodal strategies reduce the incidence of CPSP by using multiple therapies to reduce or prevent postoperative pain

iii) Postoperative
  - Aggressive and effective postoperative analgesia for patients with breakthrough pain
  - Patients who develop symptoms suggestive of neuropathic pain are being treated with agents like gabapentin. The long-term effects on CPSP are as yet unknown.

Notes

References

Haase O, Schwenk W, Hermann C, Müller JM. Guided imagery and relaxation in conventional colorectal resections: a randomized, controlled, partially blinded trial. *Diseases of the Colon and Rectum*, **48**: 1955–63, 2005

Searle RD, Simpson KH. Chronic post-surgical pain. *Continuing Education in Anaesthesia, Critical Care & Pain*, **10**: 12–14, 2010

http://www.postoppain.org (accessed 23 January 2010)

Q3 Complex Regional Pain Syndrome

a) **Outline the signs and symptoms which support a diagnosis of complex regional pain syndrome (CRPS) (9 marks)**

b) **Describe treatment modalities used in CRPS (11 marks)**

Aims

This is an examination classic and continues to appear in the written paper repeatedly. We have chosen to structure the first part of the answer according to different modalities. It is important that your answer includes not only possible pharmacological strategies but also all the extended services provided through a chronic pain team.

a) Signs and Symptoms

- Ongoing pain disproportionate to original insult or injury
- One sign present from ≥2 subsets below
- One symptom from each subset below

i) Sensory:
  - Signs: allodynia, hyperalgesia
  - Symptoms: hyperaesthesia

ii) Motor/trophic
  - Signs and symptoms: decreased range of movement, weakness, skin, hair, or nail changes

iii) Sudomotor:
  - Signs and symptoms: hyper- or hypo-hydrosis, asymmetry in sweating and/or oedema

iv) Vasomotor
  - Signs and symptoms: changes in skin colour, asymmetry in skin colour and/or temperature

b) CRPS Treatment

- Aims are to provide symptomatic pain relief and improve daily life

i) Pharmacological
  - Simple analgesia (e.g. paracetamol, NSAIDs)
  - Opioids
  - Antidepressants, anticonvulsants
  - Calcitonin (beneficial evidence not confirmed)
  - Free radical scavengers:?↓ inflammatory tissue damage (e.g. vitamin C, topical dimethylsulphoxide, IV N-acetyl-cysteine)

ii) Physical
  - Physiotherapy to improve function and limit pain
  - Motor imagery training (e.g. mirror usage): to correct inappropriate cortical remapping
  - TENS: non-invasive neuromodulation

iii) Regional Techniques
  - Intrathecal drug administration (e.g. opioids, clonidine)
  - Preoperative pre-emptive regional anaesthesia: lowers incidence and recurrence of CRPS
  - Regional nerve blockade, e.g. brachial or lumbar plexus (consider catheter and infusion)

- Sympathetic blockade:
  - IVRA (e.g. guanethidine or LA block to limb)
  - Stellate ganglion block (LA or neurolytics)

iv) Surgical Techniques
  - Thoracic or lumbar sympathectomy
  - Spinal cord stimulation: implanted epidural electrode system
  - Limb amputation: last resort for irreversible infection or ischaemia

v) Psychological
  - May be somatoform if exaggerated symptoms or signs
  - Be aware of yellow flags (i.e. anorexia, bulimia) and consider psychological review

Notes

Reference

Bush D. Complex regional pain syndrome. In: Bennett MI, ed. *Neuropathic Pain: Oxford Pain Management Library.* Oxford University Press, 2006; 57–66

Q4 Fibromyalgia

a) Define fibromyalgia (7 marks)

b) Outline different methods of treating this process (13 marks)

Aims

This condition is increasingly being managed by chronic pain teams and has been the subject of recent reviews in anaesthetic literature, both of which make it a likely topic to be included in future examination questions.

a) Definition

i) First Criteria
  * History of chronic spontaneous widespread pain for a continuous period of >3 months, including three key clinical features
    * Pain: diffuse, deep throbbing, variable intensity
    * Fatigue: worst in mornings, peaking again in early afternoon (overlap with chronic fatigue syndrome)
    * Sleep disturbance: difficulty in initiating and maintaining sleep, with frequent wakening
  * May also include:
    * morning stiffness, post-exercise pain, skin tenderness
    * tension- or migraine-like headaches, dizziness
    * paraesthesia
    * restless legs, mood disturbance
    * fluid retention

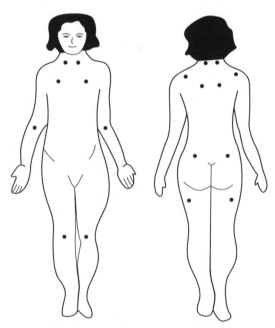

Figure 49. Fibromyalgia tenderness points

ii) Second Criteria
- Classification by American College of Rheumatology (1990)
  - Bilateral pain distribution
  - Pain above and below the waist, with axial skeleton pain present
  - Tenderness elicited upon digital palpation of 11 of 18 defined points

b) Treatment Options

- Aim is to decrease symptoms and improve quality of life
- i) General Measures
  - Patient education about awareness of the condition and its chronicity
  - Encourage a positive outlook and to remain as active as possible
  - Patient ownership of the condition
  - Introduction to patient support groups
- ii) Specific Therapies
  - Oral pharmacological
  - Standard analgesia, e.g. paracetamol, NSAIDs, tramadol (minimal evidence of benefits with opioids)
  - Neurotransmitter modifiers
  - Tricyclic antidepressant
  - Anti-epileptic therapy
  - Neuromuscular blocking agents
  - Serotonin receptor blockers
  - Monoamine oxidase inhibitors
  - Hypnotics
  - Benzodiazepines
  - Trigger point injections:
    - mixtures of local anaesthetic ± steroid have been shown to be of benefit in the short and medium term
  - IV therapy:
    - lidocaine either as a bolus (3–5mg/kg) or an infusion to block disordered pain processing pathways
  - Non-pharmacological therapy
  - Exercise and warm baths
  - Psychological assessment and treatment (e.g. cognitive behavioural therapy, health anxiety, relaxation, mindfulness)
  - Complementary therapy:
    - acupuncture
    - TENS
    - hydrotherapy

Notes

....

....

....

....

....

....

....

....

....

....

....

....

References

Dedhia JD, Bone ME. Pain and fibromyalgia. *Continuing Education in Anaesthesia, Critical Care & Pain*, **9**: 162–6, 2009

Wolfe F, Smythe HA, Yunus MB, *et al.* The American College of Rheumatology 1990 Criteria for the Classification of Fibromyalgia. Report of the Multicenter Criteria Committee. *Arthritis and Rheumatism*, **33**: 160–72, 1990

Q5 Pain Management Programme

a) **What is a pain management programme? (3 marks)**

b) **Which staff are necessary to provide a pain management programme? (3 marks)**

c) **What exclusion criteria exist for a pain management programme? (3 marks)**

d) **What are i) the educational aims (6 marks) and ii) the practical aspects (5 marks) of a pain management programme?**

Aims

Questions along these lines initially seem impossible to answer unless you have explicitly revised this topic. However, closer inspection reveals that the details are probably facts that you already know but would not initially associate with the original stem. Structures such as these often work well as templates for tackling more obscure questions that initially cause heartsink!

a) Definition

- A multifactorial programme which aims to restore the lives of chronic non-cancer pain sufferers to as close to normal as possible
- Aim is improvement of the physical, psychological, emotional, and social dimensions of the quality of life of individuals
- Use of a multidisciplinary team working according to behavioural and cognitive principles

b) Core Staff

- A medically qualified person, ideally a consultant with an interest in pain management. May be any clinician with appropriate training
- Chartered clinical psychologist or a registered cognitive behavioural therapist
- Registered physiotherapist
- Other: occupational therapist, nurses, pharmacists, clerical staff, role model patient

c) Exclusion Criteria

- Limited life expectancy or rapidly deteriorating clinical condition
- Severe psychiatric disorders affecting cognition and social behaviour
- Unresolved or untreated substance or alcohol abuse
- Physical disability such that participation in the programme is not possible

d) Aims of a Pain Management Programme

i) Educational Aims
   - To teach and aid understanding of the anatomy and physiology of pain mechanisms
   - To address psychological aspects (safety, fear, stress, depression, avoidance)
   - To provide awareness of the health and safety issues with regard to stepping up activity levels
   - Use of exercise to improve health and functional abilities
   - Advice regarding the use of remedies and drugs
   - Training in dealing with setbacks and worsening symptoms
   - To provide psychological exercises in methods of thought, emotions, and behaviour; including the use of cognitive therapies and target-setting
   - Organizing goal-directed activity using a graded approach

- Use of reinforcement to help change thought processes
- To teach exercises to improve quality and duration of sleep patterns

ii) Practical Aspects
  - Take advice from staff, practice at home, review practice, ↑ performance at controlled rate
  - Graded regular exercise
  - Graded return to goal-related activities (e.g. self-care, social activities, sport)
  - Cognitive behavioural methods to identify and challenge commonly held myths or beliefs
  - Relaxation exercises to aid sleep and enhance attention span
  - Working on communication skills with family, friends, and colleagues

Notes

Reference

British Pain Society. *Recommended Guidelines for Pain Management Programmes for Adults.* London: British Pain Society, 2007

Q6 **Pain Pathways**

a) Describe the pathway taken when a painful stimulus is administered to the sole of the foot (20 marks)

Aims

This is a very dry anatomy question which requires a certain level of detail and knowledge to be able to pass. A well-drawn clear and concise diagram can complement your written answer and shorten the time taken. However, it should not be used as a solitary method.

a) Pain Pathway

- Sensory nociceptors in skin detect painful stimulus. Primary nociceptors are free unmyelinated nerve endings which have a threshold which is exceeded to initiate an action potential
- Local tissue inflammation lowers the threshold of these receptors and activates quiescent nociceptors in adjacent tissue

  i) Peripheral
    - Primary afferent to spinal cord via two possible routes
      - Sharp fast immediate pain via myelinated A–δ fibres
        - 2–5μm diameter, conduction velocity 15–30m/sec
      - Burning diffuse unpleasant pain via unmyelinated C-fibres
        - 0.5–1.2μm diameter, conduction velocity 0.5–2m/sec
    - Cell bodies for these neurons lie in the dorsal root ganglion
    - Synapse with second-order interneurons in the dorsal horn of the spinal cord
    - A–δ fibres synapse in laminae 1 and 5
    - C-fibres synapse in substantia gelatinosa (laminae 1 and 2)
    - Some projections to inhibitory interneurons within the spinal cord
    - Fibres decussate to the contralateral side of the spinal cord

  ii) Central
    - Fibres ascend via the lateral spinothalamic tract, located in the ventrolateral quadrant of the spinal cord, to project to the thalamus
    - A small component of C-fibres ascend the cord in the spinoreticular tract
    - In the thalamus, discrimination of modality occurs according to where it synapses

    Fast Pain Spinothalamic Tract
    - Axons terminate in three main areas: ventral posterolateral nucleus (VPLN), ventral posteromedial nucleus (VPMN), and posterior nucleus (PON), collectively known as the ventroposterior nucleus
    - Associated with conscious pain perception and discrimination of differing modalities

    Slow Pain Spinothalamic Tract
    - Axons synapse with non-specific intralaminar nuclei (ILN) of the thalamus and the reticular formation in the brainstem
    - Axons are associated with affective quality of pain (unpleasantness and fear of further injury)
    - The spinoreticular pathway joins these areas
    - The VP nucleus projects third-order neurons to the cortical areas associated with pain perception
    - It displays a somatotrophic organization and third-order neurons project to a specific area of the primary sensory cortex in the parietal lobe

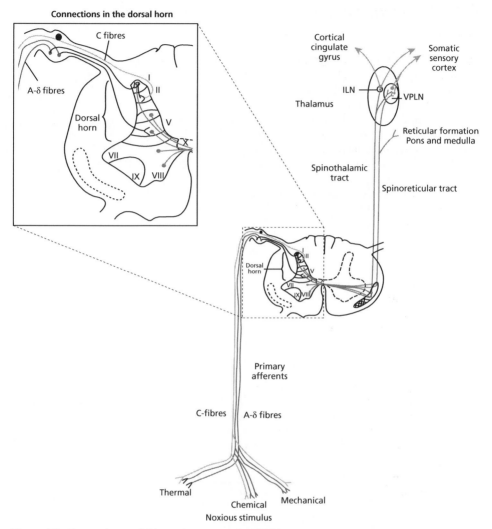

Figure 50. Pain pathways: ILN, intralaminar nuclei; VPLN, ventroposterolateral nucleus

- Slow pain impulses within the intralaminar nuclei have multiple projections:
  - anterior part of the cingulate gyrus (emotion)
  - amygdala (memory and emotion)
  - hypothalamus (emotion and the vascular response to emotion)
iii) Other Pathways Involved
Dorsal Column Pathway
- Transmits visceral nociception to the thalamus
Spinomesencephalic Pathway
- Projects to periaqueductal grey and superior colliculus linking to central areas involved in affect of pain perception

Spinohypothalamic Pathway
- Passes directly through the midbrain without synapsing to convey emotional pain information
- Multiple neurotransmitters (NTs) are involved in transmission of this impulse:
  - Excitatory: glutamate, aspartate, AMPA, calcitonin-G-related peptide, and substance P
  - Dorsal horn receptors: NMDA, opioid, adenosine, and noradrenaline

iv) Descending Inhibition
- Projections from the ascending pathways are responsible for descending inhibition of pain transmission at the spinal cord level:
  - periaqueductal grey and periventricular grey project to the nucleus raphe magnus
  - enkephalin NT activates serotoninergic descending neurons to activate inhibitory interneurons in the cord
  - Locus coeruleus has direct projection to the cord, using noradrenaline to activate inhibitory neurons

Notes

Q7 **Phantom Limb Pain**

A 65-year-old man is complaining of worsening pain 2 days post above-knee amputation of the left leg, despite an adequate PCA prescription and simple analgesia delivery.

a) What signs and symptoms suggest the development of phantom limb pain? (3 marks)

b) List the risk factors likely to increase the chances of developing phantom limb pain (5 marks)

c) Outline potential perioperative management options for this condition (12 marks)

Aims

This is a common 'on-call' scenario and may be extremely challenging to manage. The potential for developing phantom limb pain can influence anaesthetic technique, and involvement of the acute and chronic pain team is mandatory in these cases.

a) Clinical Signs and Symptoms
- Varying developmental phase, ranging from immediately post procedure to days, weeks, months, and even years afterwards
- May be induced or exacerbated by central neuraxial blockade, despite a previous asymptomatic period
- Neuropathic features (e.g. shooting, stabbing, burning, aching) may also be associated with stump pain
- Location usually at the distal end of the phantom limb
- Variation in intensity and duration from person to person; some improve to the point of cessation, while others experience constant pain which may worsen over time

b) Risk Factors
- Greater with lower than with upper limb amputation
- Greater if pre-amputation pain present
- Greater if bilateral limb amputations
- Greater if persistent stump pain exists

c) Management
i) Perioperative Analgesic Techniques
- Evidence for the success of this approach is not clear or of sufficient quality
- Methods used aim to prevent 'reprogramming' of the central nervous system which probably occurs during a prolonged course of preoperative pain
- Techniques include central neuraxial blockade (e.g. epidural infusions), combined spinal–epidural blocks, and peripheral nerve blockade or catheters (e.g. sciatic nerve blocks)

ii) Pharmacological Methods
- For postoperative pain (using the WHO pain ladder): regular paracetamol, NSAIDs (if not contraindicated), weak opioids (e.g. codeine phosphate), and strong opioids (e.g. morphine or fentanyl PCA, oxycontin, or oxynorm)

- For neuropathic phantom pain: combination of tricyclic antidepressants (TCA) (e.g. amitriptyline), anticonvulsants (e.g. gabapentin/pregabalin), and opioids used in stepwise manner:
  - either TCA or anticonvulsant
  - then TCA + anticonvulsant
  - then TCA + anticonvulsant + opioid
- Use of a lidocaine patch over the stump

iii) Physical Methods
  - Mirror box usage helps reverse the 'clenching' sensation experienced in the phantom limb
  - Acupuncture
  - Hot, cold, or massage treatments
  - TENS
  - Stump manipulation

iv) Psychological Methods
  - Cognitive behavioural therapy
  - Hypnotherapy
  - Psychotherapy
  - Educational techniques (e.g. pain management programmes)

v) Surgical
  - Excision of neuroma; considered once only
  - MicroDREZotomy (Dorsal Root Entry Zone): destruction of sensory root fibres at entry point to spinal cord and of superficial layers of dorsal horn of spinal grey matter
    - Used as last-resort procedure because of high risk of motor or sensory deficit and significant pain postoperatively

Notes

Reference

Jackson MA, Simpson KH. Pain after amputation. *Continuing Education in Anaesthesia, Critical Care & Pain*, **4**, 20–3, 2004

Q8 Transcutaneous Electrical Nerve Stimulation (TENS)

a) Describe the set-up of transcutaneous electrical nerve stimulation (TENS) and its proposed mechanism of action (8 marks)

b) Which patients may benefit from TENS? (4 marks)

c) List the contraindications to using TENS and highlight clinical scenarios where caution in its use must be adhered to (8 marks)

Aims

Concrete evidence from trials and meta-analyses on the efficacy and benefits of TENS is often lacking, but there are many anecdotal and individual stories of success. Candidates are exposed to TENS use on the labour ward and during chronic pain modules, and must be aware of application and limitations of this technique

a) TENS

- Delivery of pulsed electrical currents across intact skin surface to stimulate underlying A–β fibres
- Uses a portable battery-operated generator to deliver pulsed currents via connecting leads to self-adhering electrode conducting pads
- Self-operated by patient at home or in hospital, preferably after a supervised trial by trained nurses. The strength and frequency of pulsation is also self-controlled
- Pulse durations of 50–200µsec at 1–200 pulses/sec in a biphasic pulsed pattern
- May be used at low (1–2Hz) or high (45–150Hz) frequencies according to need
- Stimulation of large-diameter A–β fibres inhibits activity of second-order nociceptor neurons in the dorsal horn of the spinal cord via Melzack and Wall's 'gate theory'
- Stimulation of smaller-diameter A–δ fibres inhibits descending nociceptive pain pathways, activates descending inhibitory pathways (from periaqueductal grey matter and ventromedial medulla), and blocks peripheral nociceptive impulses
- Neurotransmitter release (e.g. opioids, $5HT_3$, acetyl choline, GABA, aspartate, and glutamate) may be modulated by use of high- or low-frequency TENS

b) Benefits

- Labour analgesia: placed on the back at the level corresponding to pain during the first and second stages of labour
- Postoperative pain, nausea and vomiting: some evidence of benefits over placebo
- May be used for varying forms of chronic pain (e.g. neuropathic)
- Other pain conditions (e.g. fractured ribs, lower back pain, and angina)

c) Contraindications

- Lack of knowledge or understanding of use of device
- Placement on infected, inflamed, broken, or anaesthetic skin
- Placement over the anterior portion of the neck may stimulate laryngospasm or a vagal response (e.g. bradycardia, hypotension)
- Usage in epileptics on the head or neck area may induce seizures
- Usage directly on the eyes will increase intraocular pressure

- Patients with cardiac pacemakers should be sent to cardiology for assessment and trial of TENS under directly monitored observation
- Anteroposterior placement on thorax may inhibit ventilation due to excessive stimulation of intercostal muscles
- Placement over the anterior portion of the abdomen during pregnancy may stimulate labour, or potentially affect fetal development
- Placement over ischaemic, necrotic, or thrombotic tissue may induce emboli formation
- Placement over areas with recent haemorrhage may induce further haemorrhage

Notes

References

Jones I, Johnson MI. Transcutaneous electrical nerve stimulation. *Continuing Education in Anaesthesia, Critical Care & Pain*, **9**: 130–5, 2009
Melzack R, Wall PD. Pain mechanisms: a new theory. *Science*, **150**: 971–9, 1965

Q9 Trigeminal Neuralgia

a) Define trigeminal neuralgia and describe its clinical features (4 marks)

b) Outline the risk factors and how it may be diagnosed (7 marks)

c) Discuss treatment options of the above condition (9 marks)

Aims

This question begins with a definition, often best answered with a short sentence followed by sections that lend themselves to bullet point list style answers. This can save valuable time during the examination and makes your answer relatively easier for the examiner to mark.

a) Definition and Clinical Features

- Episodic neuropathic pain described over the distribution of the trigeminal nerve
- Often associated with spasm of the muscles of mastication
- Pain: unilateral, severe, paroxysmal, lancing. 'The worst pain imaginable'
- Can affect all three branches of the trigeminal nerve, although the mandibular and maxillary branches are most common, with the ophthalmic branch involved in only 3% of cases
- May develop trigger points and allodynia (e.g. shaving in men is a classical example)

b) Risk Factors and Diagnosis

i) Risk Factors
- Female:male ratio 2:1
- Advanced age, peak onset age 60–70 years
- Hypertension
- Multiple sclerosis: most patients presenting aged between 20 and 40 years represent brainstem demyelination
- Exact aetiology remains unclear; it can follow trauma to peripheral nerves
- Current opinion points towards a vascular malformation around the trigeminal ganglion causing compression demyelination
- Central theories focus around abnormal neurons in the pons and midbrain spontaneously firing

ii) Diagnosis
- Mainly from the history
- Imaging can help to exclude brainstem lesions and vascular malformations (contrast-enhanced high resolution MRI)
- Exclusion of alternative aetiologies if the history is suggestive (e.g. post-herpetic neuralgia, multiple sclerosis, atypical facial pain, temporomandibular joint arthropathy)

c) Management

i) Pharmacological therapy
- Carbamazepine is so successful that some consider that failure to respond should prompt reinvestigation of the diagnosis. However, severe side effects exist, e.g. LFT derangement, pancytopenia, Stevens–Johnson syndrome)
- Works as maintenance and for breakthrough pain relief
- Second-line therapy includes gabapentin and lamotrigine. Other anti-epileptics are currently under investigation

- Phenytoin has benefit in patients with atypical symptoms or poor response to initial therapy
- Baclofen may help with spasm: dose of 60–80mg although evidence is divided; L-baclofen appears to be more effective

ii) Surgical therapy
- Indicated in patients with poor response to medical therapy or young age of onset
- Percutaneous trans-sphenoidal procedures (e.g. balloon decompression or pulsed radiofrequency ablation of ganglion).
  - Works almost immediately
  - Shortest pain free period, usually 1–4 years
  - Reserved for elderly patients with shorter life expectancy where a poor tolerance of craniotomy would be expected
- Gamma knife techniques
  - Can take months to provide benefit
  - Stereotactic-guided radio-ablation
  - More consistent results than percutaneous techniques
  - Less risk of nerve injury compared with open surgical procedures
- Open decompression
  - Requires GA and posterior cranial fossa exploration; often long surgery
  - Microvascular decompression and ablation of anomalies
  - Can provide pain relief for upwards of 15 years
  - Risks nerve injury, subsequent dysthesia, and complete anaesthesia of the face (incidence 15%)

Notes

References

Broggi GP, Ferroli P, Franzini A, Servello D, Dones I. Microvascular decompression for trigeminal neuralgia: comments on a series of 250 cases, including 10 patients with multiple sclerosis. *Journal of Neurology, Neurosurgery and Psychiatry*, **68**: 59–64, 2000

http://emedicine.medscape.com/article/1145144-treatment (accessed 13 October 2009)

Index

Index